Problem and Pathological Gambling

James P. Whelan
Gambling Clinic and The Institute for Gambling Education and
Research at The University of Memphis, Memphis, TN

Timothy A. Steenbergh
Department of Psychology, Indiana Wesleyan University, Marion, IN

Andrew W. Meyers
Gambling Clinic and The Institute for Gambling Education and
Research at The University of Memphis, Memphis, TN

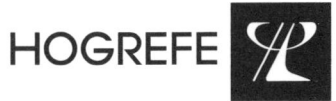

Library of Congress Cataloging in Publication

is available via the Library of Congress Marc Database under the
LC Control Number 2007922289

RC
569.5
.G35
W44
2007

Library and Archives Canada Cataloguing in Publication

Whelan, James P.
    Problem and pathological gambling / James P. Whelan, Timothy A. Steenbergh, Andrew W. Meyers.

(Advances in psychotherapy – evidence-based practice)
Includes bibliographical references.
ISBN 978-0-88937-312-9

    1. Compulsive gambling. 2. Compulsive gambling – Treatment. 3. Compulsive gamblers – Rehabilitation. I. Steenbergh, Timothy A. II. Meyers, Andrew W., 1949- III. Title. IV. Series.
HV6710.W48 2007   616.85'841   C2007-900942-5

© 2007 by Hogrefe & Huber Publishers

PUBLISHING OFFICES
USA: Hogrefe & Huber Publishers, 875 Massachusetts Avenue, 7th Floor, Cambridge, MA 02139
Phone (866) 823-4726, Fax (617) 354-6875; E-mail info@hhpub.com
EUROPE: Hogrefe & Huber Publishers, Rohnsweg 25, 37085 Göttingen, Germany
Phone +49 551 49609-0, Fax +49 551 49609-88, E-mail hh@hhpub.com

SALES & DISTRIBUTION
USA: Hogrefe & Huber Publishers, Customer Services Department,
30 Amberwood Parkway, Ashland, OH 44805
Phone (800) 228-3749, Fax (419) 281-6883, E-mail custserv@hhpub.com
EUROPE: Hogrefe & Huber Publishers, Rohnsweg 25, 37085 Göttingen, Germany
Phone +49 551 49609-0, Fax +49 551 49609-88, E-mail hh@hhpub.com

OTHER OFFICES
CANADA: Hogrefe & Huber Publishers, 1543 Bayview Avenue, Toronto, Ontario M4G 3B5
SWITZERLAND: Hogrefe & Huber Publishers, Länggass-Strasse 76, CH-3000 Bern 9

Hogrefe & Huber Publishers
Incorporated and registered in the State of Washington, USA, and in Göttingen, Lower Saxony, Germany

No part of this book may be reproduced, stored in a retrieval system or transmitted, in any form or by any means, electronic, mechanical, photocopying, microfilming, recording or otherwise, without written permission from the publisher.

Printed and bound in the USA
ISBN 978-0-88937-312-9

Preface

The mathematician Amir Aczel (2004) introduced his book on probability and gambling with the following statement, "The twin forces of chance and mischance have beguiled humanity like none other." Amir noted that gambling has been a common recreational activity since the earliest of human cultures. Of course, the games have changed over time. The sheep knuckle dice thrown by the early Greeks barely resemble the smooth, uniform cubes we toss across felt tables. What has remained constant is our fascination with gambling, the possibilities of winning and the threat of losing everything.

Today gambling is a vital part of many economic systems. Consider the history of gambling in the United States where there have almost always been forms of legal gambling and some amount of illegal gambling has been tolerated. In fact, lotteries were sanctioned during the American Revolution to raise revenue for the continental armies. Since that time the laws and public opinion concerning gambling in the U.S. have cycled to allow and then contain gambling. The most recent widespread legalization of gambling began in 1970. Twenty years later, the gross gambling revenue from legal forms of gambling was reported to be 73 billion U.S. dollars. By 2006 some form of legalized gambling was available in every state other than Utah and Hawaii, with 43 states running their own lotteries. Despite the availability of legalized forms of gambling, illegal gambling still exists and, by some accounts, flourishes in the U.S.

Some of the hoped for economic benefits to the communities with legal gambling has occurred. Revenues from state lotteries fund a variety of social support activities, including public education, public housing, health care programs, transportation, senior citizen programs, and property tax decreases. It has been argued that continued government support for these social programs relies on gambling revenue. For example, Hurricane Katrina in 2005 eliminated 13 casinos along the state's Gulf of Mexico coast. The state of Mississippi reported losing approximately $500,000 per day in tax revenue and the governor hurriedly called a special legislative session in order to encourage casino corporations to rebuild in the region.

The recent expansion in gambling availability has been fueled by the tremendous popularity of gambling as a recreational activity. In 1999 and 2000, Welte and colleagues (Welte, Barnes, Wieczorek, Tidwell, & Parker, 2002) completed a random digit dialing survey of over 2,500 individuals over the age of 18 years. With this survey they collected considerable detail about respondents' gambling behavior during the previous year. The results, statistically weighted to match the U.S. census, showed that 82% of respondents had gambled during the past year and 23% gambled weekly. By way of comparison, 15% of American adults attended a live theater performance and 43% read a book during the previous year.

For most people gambling offers a fantasy we may not be able to create in any other way. As we pull the handle on the slot machine, push the poker chips to the middle of a table, or pick the lucky number of the multimillion dollar lottery, we wonder what we would do if we won more money than we could earn in a week, a year, or many lifetimes. Regrettably, the cost of misfortune can be destructive. What helps us to understand the homemaker who slips off to the casino as soon as her children leave for school? Why does she believe that she will soon win enough money to replenish her children's education fund? What about the 41-year-old restaurant manager who skims money from daily receipts in order to bankroll his next poker game? Can we make sense of the accountant who takes the $500 remaining in his checking account to place bets on next weekend's football games in the hope of paying off his $1,200 credit card bill? For some, gambling is clearly more than risking money on a game of chance.

Like Aczel's book, ours focuses on playing games of chance and the experience of luck. Unlike Aczel, our interest is in how to provide assistance to those who have been captivated and then seriously harmed by gambling. In the first three chapters of this book we provide background information about problem and pathological gambling, current models for understanding these problems, and information we believe is relevant for assessment and treatment. Chapter 4 presents details about using our treatment for gambling problems, "Guided Self-Change for Gambling." This is followed in Chapter 5 with a presentation of a gambler who presented in our treatment clinic. The final chapters of the book provide other tools and information that you might find helpful. We hope by reading this book you gain an understanding of gambling behavior, the problems it can produce, and guidelines for effectively treating problematic gambling.

Acknowledgments

There are a number of people that we would like to acknowledge as valuable contributors to this project. First we thank Danny Wedding and Robert Dimbleby for their guidance, patience, and support. We would also like to thank our former and current graduate students for their creative input in our discussions about gambling, our understanding about gambling problems, and our success as a research team. In particular, we thank Ryan May for his enthusiastic insights as we developed and piloted our treatment. We also thank Damon Lipinski for his careful attention to detail and his willingness to take on all challenges. The other bright minds who made valuable contributions include: Angie Sheffield, Kim Floyd, Jeremiah Weinstock, Emerson Wickwire, Andrea Booth, Adrienne Studaway, Don Yorgason, Rebecca West, and Claudia McClausland. We also appreciate the efforts of Brian Fry for his feedback on early drafts. Finally, we are greatly indebted to Linda and Mark Sobell. Their pioneering efforts to treat addictive behavior and their tireless dedication to the science of clinical psychology have been inspiring. In particular, Linda's generous support in helping us learn how to think about addiction and gambling problems has been instrumental to our work.

Dedication

We would like to dedicate this book to our families.
  Ginger, Ellen, and Zoe Whelan
  Tracey, Jackson, and Molley Steenbergh
  Lee, Brian, and Abby Meyers

Table of Contents

Preface v
Acknowledgments vi
Dedication vii

1 Description of Problem and Pathological Gambling 1
1.1   Terminology 1
1.1.1 Gambling as Recreation 1
1.1.2 Continuum of Gambling-Related Harm 2
1.2   Definitions 4
1.2.1 Pathological Gambling 4
1.2.2 Problem Gambling 6
1.3   Epidemiology 7
1.3.1 Vulnerable Populations 7
1.3.2 Types of Gambling and Gambling Problems 9
1.3.3 Impact of Gambling Availability 9
1.3.4 Demographic Correlates 10
1.4   Course and Prognosis 11
1.4.1 Negative Effects 12
1.4.2 Natural Recovery 12
1.5   Differential Diagnosis 13
1.6   Comorbidity 13
1.6.1 Substance Use Disorders 13
1.6.2 Mood Disorders 14
1.6.3 Anxiety Disorders 15
1.6.4 Axis II Disorders 15
1.7   Diagnostic Procedures and Documentation 15
1.7.1 Diagnostic Interview for Gambling Severity (DIGS) 15
1.7.2 South Oaks Gambling Screen (SOGS) 16
1.7.3 Lie/Bet Questionnaire 16
1.7.4 Gambling Timeline Follow-Back (G-TLFB) 16
1.7.5 Addiction Severity Index – Gambling Subscale (ASI-G) . . 17
1.7.6 Gamblers Belief Questionnaire (GBQ) 18
1.7.7 Gamblers Self-Efficacy Questionnaire (GSEQ) 18

2 Theories and Models 20
2.1   Gambling as an Addictive Behavior 20
2.2   Learning Theories 22
2.3   Cognitive Theories 24
2.4   Biological Theories 27
2.4.1 Family and Genetic Studies 27
2.4.2 Neurotransmitter and Neuroanatomical Theories 28
2.5   Disease Model 29
2.6   An Integrated Model of Problem Gambling 30
2.7   Guided Self-Change 31

2.7.1	Harm Reduction	32
2.7.2	Rapid Change Response	32
2.7.3	Self-Change	33
2.7.4	Motivational Approach	34

3 Diagnosis and Treatment Indications ... 35
- 3.1 Diagnostic Assessment ... 35
- 3.2 Treatment Indications ... 35
- 3.3 Clinical Assessment ... 36
- 3.3.1 Gambling Behavior ... 37
- 3.3.2 Assessment of Possible Treatment Mediators ... 37
- 3.3.3 Systemic Factors ... 39
- 3.3.4 Comorbid Psychopathology ... 40
- 3.4 Treatments ... 41

4 Treatment ... 43
- 4.1 Method of Treatment ... 43
- 4.1.1 Basic Principles ... 43
- 4.1.2 Phase 1: Running Start Assessment ... 47
- 4.1.3 Phase 2: Motivational Feedback ... 49
- 4.1.4 Phase 3: Triggers and Consequences ... 52
- 4.1.5 Phase 4: Options and Action Plan ... 53
- 4.1.6 Phase 5: Relapse Prevention ... 55
- 4.1.7 Follow-Up ... 56
- 4.2 Mechanisms of Action ... 57
- 4.3 Efficacy and Diagnosis ... 58
- 4.4 Variations and Combination Methods ... 59
- 4.5 Problems in Carrying Out Treatment ... 61
- 4.6 Multicultural Issues ... 62

5 Case Vignette ... 64
- 5.1 Phase 1: Running Start Assessment ... 64
- 5.2 Phase 2: Motivation and Feedback ... 68
- 5.3 Phase 3: Functional Analysis of Gambling ... 76
- 5.4 Phase 4: Implementation of Alternative Behaviors ... 78
- 5.5 Phase 5: Relapse Prevention ... 79
- 5.6 Six Month Follow-up ... 80

6 Further Reading ... 82

7 References ... 83

8 Appendices: Tools and Resources ... 91

Problem and Pathological Gambling

About the Authors

James P. Whelan, PhD, is Associate Professor of Psychology and Director of Clinical Training at the University of Memphis, as well as codirector of the Institute for Gambling Education and Research and the Gambling Clinic. He has also served as Director of Clinical Training and has won awards for his engaged scholarship. Dr. Whelan's research spans several areas, including efficacy for psychological treatments, problem gambling, and sport and exercise psychology.

Timothy A. Steenbergh, PhD, is Associate Professor of Psychology and Director of the Lilly Student Research Initiative at Indiana Wesleyan University. Dr. Steenbergh's research on addictive behaviors has focused primarily on problem gambling. In addition to his research, Dr. Steenbergh also enjoys teaching and providing psychotherapy at a small clinical practice in Marion, IN.

Andrew W. Meyers, PhD, is Professor in the Department of Psychology and Vice Provost for Research at the University of Memphis, as well as codirector of the Institute for Gambling Education and Research. Dr. Meyers has served on the editorial boards of the *Journal of Consulting and Clinical Psychology*, *Behavior Therapy*, *Health Psychology*, and *Cognitive Therapy and Research*, and for the past 25 years has maintained a private practice focused on addictions and health behavior.

Advances in Psychotherapy – Evidence-Based Practice

Danny Wedding; PhD, MPH, Prof., St. Louis, MO
(Series Editor)
Larry Beutler; PhD, Prof., Palo Alto, CA
Kenneth E. Freedland; PhD, Prof., St. Louis, MO
Linda C. Sobell; PhD, ABPP, Prof., Ft. Lauderdale, FL
David A. Wolfe; PhD, Prof., Toronto
(Associate Editors)

The basic objective of this series is to provide therapists with practical, evidence-based treatment guidance for the most common disorders seen in clinical practice – and to do so in a "reader-friendly" manner. Each book in the series is both a compact "how-to-do" reference on a particular disorder for use by professional clinicians in their daily work, as well as an ideal educational resource for students and for practice-oriented continuing education.
The most important feature of the books is that they are practical and "reader-friendly." All are structured similarly and all provide a compact and easy-to-follow guide to all aspects that are relevant in real-life practice. Tables, boxed clinical "pearls," marginal notes, and summary boxes assist orientation, while checklists provide tools for use in daily practice.

1

Description of Problem and Pathological Gambling

1.1 Terminology

Gambling can be defined as any behavior involving the risk of money or valuable possessions on the outcome of a game, contest, or other event in which the outcome is at least partially determined by chance. There are many forms of gambling: purchasing lottery tickets, participating in sports pools, an evening at the casino, wagers on the golf course, or speculating on the futures and stock markets. Sometimes we actually call it gambling; other times we use terms that are less pejorative, such as gaming, investing, or a friendly wager.

Gambling defined

A variety of terminology has been used to describe the degree to which individuals experience gambling-related problems. Some of these terms, such as compulsive gambling, reflect dated conceptualizations of the problem while others were adopted as early screening instruments were developed. Understanding this language can be difficult, particularly because many of the terms have been used inconsistently. We will return to this issue in Section 1.1.2.

1.1.1 Gambling as Recreation

The study by Welte and colleagues (2002) has provided a great deal of information about the gambling behavior of those living in the U.S. As shown in Table 1, individuals who have gambled in the past year wagered an average of $1,735 over 60 episodes during that year. While similar percentages of women and men gambled, interesting differences between the two emerge. Compared to women, men were more likely to gamble weekly, wager more frequently, and with more money. A smaller percentage of ethno-cultural minorities, compared to Caucasians, gambled, but if they did gamble they tended to gamble more often and spend more money. The percentage of respondents who gambled in the past year decreased with increasing age. However, the amount of money wagered per year did not change as age increased. Gamblers wagered with similar frequency and intensity regardless of age.

Gambling is available and acceptable

Purchasing lottery tickets (66%) was by far the most common form of gambling followed by raffles, charitable gambling, or office pools (48%). However the level of financial investment in these activities was considerably lower than for other forms of gambling. Twenty-seven percent of respondents reported casino gambling. Casino gamblers, racetrack bettors, and dice game players tended to expend larger amounts of money compared to those who engaged in other gambling activities. Interestingly, internet gambling was reported by less

Table 1
Past Year Gambling as Reported in the National Survey on Gambling Behavior, 1999–2000 (N = 2630)

	% Gambled	% Gambled weekly	Mean gambling episodes	Mean gambling involvement in U.S.$/yr.
All	82	23	60	$1,735
Sex				
Female	80	17	46	$1,097
Male	84	29	74	$2,390
Ethnicity				
Caucasian	83	23	54	$1,295
African-American	75	26	97	$3,763
Hispanic	83	22	65	$2,223
Asian-American	82	16	37	$1,379
Age				
18–30 yrs	89	19	53	$1,689
31–40 yrs	86	25	63	$1,729
41–50 yrs	83	28	60	$2,052
51–60 yrs	81	28	66	$1,559
61+ yrs	69	21	63	$1,582

Adapted from Welte, J. W., Barnes, G. M., Weiczorek, W. F., Tidwell, M. C., & Parker, J. (2002). Gambling participation in the U.S.: Results from a national survey. *Journal of Gambling Studies, 18*, 313–338.

than one percent of the sample, although most believe that internet gambling is a growing market, and possibly a growing problem.

For those living on the U.S. mainland, casinos are within a few hours drive of their home or work, lottery tickets are a corner store away, and internet gambling can be readily accessed on the home or office computer. This provides easy access to a leisure activity that continues to enjoy growing acceptance.

1.1.2 Continuum of Gambling-Related Harm

Gambling problems have been around as long as gambling itself and many professionals have explored the psychology behind this problematic behavior. Accompanying the recent proliferation of legalized gambling has been an increasing push to refine how gambling-related problems are conceptualized. The view that has dominated the treatment and research literature in recent years is that gambling-related harm exists on a continuum from no gambling to severe problems or pathological gambling (National Research Council, 1999; Shaffer, Hall, & Vander Bilt, 1997).

Table 2
Continuum of Gambling-Related Harm

	Category	Description	Adult lifetime prevalence (95% confidence interval)	Adult past year prevalence (95% confidence interval)
Level 1	Recreational gambler or nongambler	If gambles, it is for social reasons and rarely exceeds self-imposed limits	94.7% (93.7 to 95.6)	96.1% (95 to 97)
Level 2	Problem gambler	Some diagnostic symptoms or gambling-related distress; subclinical	3.8% (2.9 to 4.8)	2.8% (2.0 to 4.8)
Level 3	Pathological gambler	Meets at least 5 diagnostic criteria	1.7% (1.4 to 1.9)	1.1% (0.9 to 1.4)

Adapted from Shaffer, H. J., Hall, M. N., & Vander Bilt, J. (1997). *Estimating the prevalence of disordered gambling behavior in the United States and Canada: A meta-analysis.* Harvard Medical School Division of Addiction.

This continuum was initially proposed as an attempt to organize the confusing and chaotic set of labels used to describe those who have been harmed by their gambling. Some of the terms that have appeared in the clinical and research literature include compulsive gambling, at-risk gambling, in-transition gambling, potentially pathological gambling, and probable pathological gambling. In an effort to organize these concepts in order to estimate the prevalence of gambling problems, Shaffer and colleagues proposed a continuum of gambling harm (see Table 2). At one end of the continuum are those who gamble for social or recreational reasons. They use their discretionary money to gamble and are reluctant to exceed their self-imposed monetary limits. These individuals, sometimes referred to as recreational gamblers or Level 1 gamblers, typically wager with little or no financial, psychological, or interpersonal harm.

Shaffer and colleagues (1997) described those in the middle of the continuum as having subclinical levels of gambling problems and defined them as Level 2 gamblers. They present some gambling-related symptoms or problems, but do not meet diagnostic criteria. Level 2 gambling is an ambiguous concept. It includes people who have reported one gambling-related problem or gambling-related symptom during the past year as well as those who might have historically had gambling concerns but currently do not meet diagnostic criteria. These individuals may be in transition toward either end of the continuum, but they might also continue to experience a modest level of gambling-related problems or symptoms for years. Their clinical manifestations, therefore, vary widely. Level 2 gamblers have been considered analogous to individuals diagnosed with substance abuse disorder.

At the far end of the continuum are those who meet criteria for pathological gambling disorder. Referred to by Shaffer and colleagues as Level 3 gamblers, they present with severe and persistent gambling-related symptoms. Their problems are seen as chronic, debilitating, and include significant impairment in daily functioning (National Research Council, 1999). Such impairment might include conflict or deterioration in relationships with spouses or significant others, loss of a home, work performance problems or job loss, and criminal involvement. Details about this diagnosis are provided below.

Although initially proposed as a method for organizing the prevalence literature, the idea of a continuum of harm has provided researchers and clinicians with a model for examining level of gambling involvement and severity of gambling problems (National Research Council, 1999; Petry, 2005a). Some have proposed using the term disordered gambling to describe both Level 2 and Level 3 gambling. To date, little research has explored how individuals progress along the continuum.

1.2 Definitions

The recent clinical and research literature has focused on two levels of gambling problems: pathological gambling (or Level 3) and problem gambling (or Level 2).

1.2.1 Pathological Gambling

An impulse control disorder with addictive symptoms

Pathological Gambling (312.31) is the diagnosis as classified in the Diagnostic and Statistical Manual of Mental Disorders, Fourth Edition – Text revision (DSM-IV-TR; American Psychiatric Association, 2000). This diagnosis is listed under the category of "Impulse Control Disorders Not Elsewhere Classified." To qualify for the diagnosis, an individual must meet five or more of the ten criteria listed in Table 3 and these symptoms must have existed at some time during the past year. There are three symptom clusters: disruption to the individual's life, loss of control, and dependence. The cut-off of five criteria was a clinical decision and has not yet been empirically validated. The course of pathological gambling is thought to be chronic.

The disorder is characterized by the gambling-related problems described in the previous section and a periodic or continuous loss of control over gambling. Impulse control disorders in general are characterized by a failure to resist an impulse to engage in some behavior, increased tension before committing the behavior, and pleasure or release following the behavior. The listing as "Not Elsewhere Classified" was initially used because gambling problems did not appear to have features beyond impulse dysregulation to aid classification. Pathological gambling was categorized as an impulse control disorder because those who gamble excessively exhibit impulsivity in their inability to stop gambling and their tendency to "chase" gambling losses. Chasing, a symptom unique to gambling, is the continuation or the initiation of a gambling session in order to recover money recently lost. Research suggests that impulsivity differentiates pathological gamblers from those who gamble recreationally (e.g., Steel & Blaszczynski, 2002). For example, indicators of behavioral disinhibi-

Table 3
Diagnostic Criteria for Pathological Gambling (312.31)

A. Persistent and recurrent maladaptive gambling behavior as indicated by five (or more) of the following:
   1. Is preoccupied with gambling (e.g., preoccupied with reliving past gambling experiences, handicapping, or planning the next venture, or thinking of ways to get money with which to gamble).
   2. Needs to gamble with increasing amounts of money in order to achieve the desired excitement.
   3. Has repeated unsuccessful efforts to control, cut back, or stop gambling
   4. Is restless or irritable when attempting to cut down or stop gambling.
   5. Gambles as a way of escaping problems or of relieving a dysphoric mood (e.g., feelings of helplessness, guilt, anxiety, depression).
   6. After losing money gambling, often returns another day to get even ("chasing" one's losses).
   7. Lies to family members, therapist, or others to conceal the extent of involvement with gambling.
   8. Has committed illegal acts such as forgery, fraud, theft, or embezzlement to finance gambling.
   9. Has jeopardized or lost a significant relationship, job, or educational or career opportunity because of gambling.
   10. Relied on others to provide money to relieve a desperate financial situation caused by gambling.

B. The gambling behavior is not better accounted for by a manic episode.

Reprinted with permission from the *Diagnostic and Statistical Manual of Mental Disorders, Fourth Edition – Text Revision*, © 2000 American Psychiatric Association.

tion – the inability to inhibit behavioral impulses – have been associated with gambling involvement and with some individuals who present with gambling problems.

The dependence cluster of symptoms appeared when the diagnostic criteria were revised (American Psychiatric Association, 1987) in response to criticism that the initial criteria placed too much emphasis on external consequences. Symptoms of dependence included increased tolerance, experience of withdrawal, and preoccupation with either the behavior or escaping from problems. Clearly, this decision reflected the growing view among treatment providers that pathological gambling appeared similar to substance dependence. Rosenthal (1989) observed that the pathological gambling criteria were essentially the substance dependence criteria with the word substance replaced by the word gambling.

Much research is needed to further understand excessive gambling. Researchers are only beginning to understand its etiology and treatment (Blaszczynski, & Nower, 2002; National Research Council, 1999; Petry, 2005a; Toneatto, 1999). The diagnosis is based on clinical description and much work is needed before we have an empirically tested model for understanding those who meet this diagnosis. It is also important to note that some potential models of excessive gambling do not require a medical model diagnosis. There is much to be said, however, for the current description of pathological gambling. The criteria are stated in precise operational terms that provide the possibility for psychometrically sound measurement tools.

1.2.2 Problem Gambling

Subclinical level of gambling problems

Problem gambling, compared to pathological gambling, is a somewhat more ambiguous term than pathological gambling and generally reflects the experience of significant gambling-related negative consequences. In recent years this term has been used as a synonym for Level 2 gambling, suggesting a subclinical level of gambling problems (Shaffer et al., 1997, 1999). Problem gamblers experience less than five of the ten symptoms of pathological gambling or their responses on gambling screening measures indicate gambling problems at a severity less than what is considered necessary for diagnostic consideration. Problem gamblers are analogous to substance abusers who receive that diagnosis as opposed to a substance dependence diagnosis. They are an understudied population (Blaszczynski, Ladouceur, & Shaffer, 2004). It remains unclear if these individuals are transitioning along the continuum from recreational gambling to pathological gambling or if they experience moderate, but chronic, negative consequences due to their gambling behavior. Petry (2005a) observed that problem gamblers might experience benefits from some reduction in their gambling, but they are also unlikely to enter into treatment. They may, however, benefit from public awareness and prevention efforts (Blaszczynski et al., 2004).

The concept of problem gambling can also be considered analogous to the term problem drinking. Both conceptions of these addictive behaviors are useful for those who do not wish to adopt a medical model that emphasizes distinct diagnostic entities. Used in this manner, the label refers to problems created when an individual continues to engage in a behavior despite the damaging or harmful consequences (e.g., Walker & Dickerson, 1996). Problem gambling, therefore, can refer to all Level 2 and Level 3 gamblers. Some problem gamblers will meet diagnostic criteria for pathological gambling and others will not. While it is likely that diagnostic symptoms are present, problem gambling is a description of behavior related to its consequences rather than a set of diagnostic criteria. One of the benefits of this perspective is that it places the focus on the problematic behavior and not on judgments of intensity. This definition of problem gambling is also consistent with literature suggesting that more intense problems do not necessarily require more intense treatments. For example, a growing body of research has found that brief treatments are effective for more severely dependent drinkers (e.g., Sobell & Sobell, 1998). Despite expectations that serious problems require lengthier, more intense treatment, these studies found that response to treatment was unrelated to treatment length or problem severity.

For this volume we use the term problem gambling to indicate anyone with a gambling-related problem. Problem gamblers include those who meet diagnostic criteria for pathological gambling, as well as those who present with problems due to their gambling but do not meet diagnostic criteria. At this time, the gambling treatment literature does not support the fact that differences in the intensity of gambling problems or differences in the type or pattern of gambling itself require different treatment approaches.

1.3 Epidemiology

As listed in Table 2, the lifetime prevalence rate for adult Level 3, or pathological gambling, is 1.7% and the past year prevalence is 1.1%. For Level 2 gambling the lifetime prevalence rate for adults is 3.8% and the past year prevalence is 2.8%. These estimates were derived from a meta-analysis of 120 prevalence studies that were available before June of 1997 (Shaffer, Hall, & Vander Bilt, 1997; 1999). These rates suggest that approximately 5.4% of the population, or about one out of 20 adults in North America, have experienced significant gambling problems in their lifetime and about 4%, or one in 25, experienced gambling problems during the past year.

Several other prevalence studies (Gerstein et al., 1999; Ladouceur, 1996; Welte, Barnes, Wieczorek, Tidwell, & Parker, 2001) have generated estimates of problem and pathological gambling reasonably consistent with the estimates presented in the prevalence meta-analysis. Gerstein and colleagues (1999) did report significantly lower prevalence estimates in their national prevalence study. These lower rates are likely due to methodological and measurement differences.

Estimates of the prevalence of gambling problems in countries outside of North America are not as well established. In general these estimates of lifetime or past year problem and pathological gambling are consistent with the prevalence meta-analysis findings. For example, the lifetime prevalence of pathological gambling in European and Asian studies appears to be between 1% and 2%. Lifetime rates of problem gambling appear to be between 2% and 5%. Estimates of past year problem and pathological gambling are approximately half the lifetime estimates.

Prevalence rates among adults

1.3.1 Vulnerable Populations

Concerns have been raised about the potential vulnerability of specific demographic subgroups to gambling-related problems (for a discussion of these concerns, see National Research Council, 1999). Membership in any of these groups seems to indicate an increased risk for gambling-related problems. The literature about identified at-risk populations has not been exhaustive and little is known about other potentially vulnerable groups.

Adolescents
While the instruments used to estimate prevalence among adolescents are not without controversy, both high school and college age adolescents appear to be particularly vulnerable to problem gambling (Derevensky, Gupta, & Winters, 2003; Shaffer & Hall, 1996; Shaffer et al., 1999). As gambling is illegal for adolescents in most jurisdictions, gambling involvement itself places adolescents at risk for legal difficulties. Between 77% and 83% of high school students report having gambled in the past year (Shaffer & Hall, 1996). About 3% to 8% of adolescents can be described as past year Level 3 gamblers and an additional 9% to 20% report past year behavior and consequences consistent with Level 2 gambling (Shaffer et al., 1999). Gambling among this age cohort has been shown to be correlated with involvement in other problem behaviors,

Heightened rates of problems among adolescents

including substance use, delinquency, and poor academic achievement (e.g., Barnes, Welte, Hoffman, & Dintcheff, 2005; Stinchfield, 2000).

While most college students have gambled during the past year, 3% to 6% of college students appear to be Level 2 gamblers and another 4% to 14% can be described as Level 3 gamblers (Engwall, Hunter, & Steinberg, 2004; Shaffer et al., 1999). When compared to Level 1 gamblers, college students with gambling problems report poorer academic performance and greater risk-taking, including heavy alcohol consumption and illicit drug use.

The high rates of problematic gambling by adolescents and college students should be interpreted with caution. We know little about how the research on adult problem and pathological gambling translates to adolescents. For example, the number of gambling symptoms reported by adolescents decreases substantially when the screening measures are modified to indicate the impact of behavioral symptoms (Ladouceur et al., 2000). For example, adolescent respondents might report that they have lied about their gambling, but also indicate that the lying had no impact on their lives. Similarly, many adolescents may gamble away all their funds, yet not jeopardize their safety and security because their parents serve as a buffer to serious consequences.

Older Adults

Low rates of problems among adults

In contrast to adolescents, adults over the age of 60 years are much less likely to be classified as Level 2 or Level 3 gamblers. For example, Welte and colleagues (2001) found that 2.2% of the respondents over the age of 61 were classified as Level 2 gamblers and 0.1% were classified as Level 3 during the past year. These findings should be viewed as preliminary since few prevalence studies have examined the gambling behavior of those over 60 and those studies have used relatively small samples. Several nonrandom samples of those over age 60 who were recruited from gambling venues have found, as expected, higher rates of problem and pathological gambling (e.g., Ladd, Molinda, Kerins, & Perry, 2003).

Substance Abusers

Substance users appear vulnerable

Individuals with a history of substance abuse appear to be particularly vulnerable to gambling problems. In their meta-analysis Shaffer et al., (1999) estimated that 15% of adults in treatment for a substance abuse disorder were identified as problem gamblers and 14% were identified as pathological gamblers during their lifetime. An increased risk for problem gambling has been found for those with general substance abuse, and among those who use alcohol, cocaine, opioids, and cannabis.

Casino Employees

Many believe that casino employees may be at risk for gambling-related problems because of their proximity and access to gambling. In a study of employees at three casinos, the rate of past year pathological gambling (2.1%) was higher and the rate of problem gambling (1.4%) lower than general population estimates (Shaffer, Vander Bilt, & Hall, 1999). A subsequent longitudinal study at six casinos found initial rates of both problem (21.2%) and pathological (4.3%) gambling to be significantly higher than general population estimates (Shaffer & Hall, 2002). This study employed relatively liberal criteria for identifying problem gambling which might explain the higher rates.

1.3.2 Types of Gambling and Gambling Problems

A subset of the prevalence reports has allowed researchers to ask about the relation between type of gambling and gambling problems. Specifically, these studies asked whether the proportion of problem and pathological gamblers among players who preferred some games was higher than the base rate predicted by the prevalence studies. Ideally, such information might reveal games that are more likely to attract problem gamblers. These studies have generally failed to identify clear differences. Approaching the issue from a different perspective, Petry and Mallya (2004) found elevated rates of problem gambling among those who had attempted to gamble on the internet or play video poker. While problems related to internet gambling have been noted in the literature, existing evidence suggests that the rate of problems due to internet gambling is surprisingly low (e.g., Ladd & Petry, 2002a).

No clear association between type of gambling and gambling problems

1.3.3 Impact of Gambling Availability

Evidence suggests the prevalence of problem gambling has increased with gambling availability (National Research Council, 1999; Petry 2003a). Shaffer and colleagues (Shaffer et al., 1999) found that the average prevalence rate of problem gambling before 1993 was 4.4% and the average prevalence rate between 1993 and 1997 was 6.7%. Studies comparing gambling before and after the introduction of new forms of legalized gambling find either a significant increase in problem gambling or no change across time (e.g., Grun & McKeigue, 2000).

Understanding the relation between gambling availability and gambling problems is not simple. Measurement and prevalence methods have changed across time and limit our ability to definitively predict the effects of greater availability on the rate of gambling problems. It is also unclear whether new gambling options in locations where gambling is already available influences problem gambling. The evolving cultural attitude toward gambling is another factor that will likely influence the relationship between availability and problems. Finally, public awareness of gambling problems might mediate the influence of availability. In their three-year study of casino employees, Shaffer and Hall (2002) found that rates of problem and pathological gambling tended to decrease over time. One possible reason for this decrease is improved awareness of gambling problems and greater support for those who have experienced problems. Considering the present state of the literature, it can be said that gambling exposure seems necessary for someone to have a gambling problem, but availability is likely to be just one of several factors that cause gambling problems.

1.3.4 Demographic Correlates

Research has identified that the following demographic variables are associated with problem gambling. Be aware that many of these demographic variables are interrelated. For example, in some communities membership in an ethnic minority group is related to socioeconomic status. In addition, the relationship between gambling problems and a demographic variable might be explained by other variables not considered in the literature. For example, it is possible that the difference in the rates of gambling problems for married and unmarried individuals might be attributable to a third variable such as social support.

Age

> Problems more common among adolescents and young adults

As noted previously, rates of gambling problems vary with age. Gambling problems are higher among adolescents and young adults than among older adults. Fourteen of the 17 general population studies that examined prevalence across age groups found that individuals below the age of 30 years were disproportionately more likely to have gambling problems (National Research Council, 1999). Prevalence studies from other jurisdictions around the world show similar results. Despite higher rates of problem gambling among youth, they appear less likely to present for treatment (Petry & Oncken, 2002; Stinchfield & Winters, 2001; Volberg, 1994).

Gender

> Men more likely to have gambling problems

Males are more likely than females to have gambling problems (Welte et al., 2001; Shaffer et al., 1999). Of 18 studies examining gender and gambling, Shaffer and colleagues (1997) found 17 reported significantly higher rates of problem gambling among males. These gender effects vary by age, with younger cohorts experiencing greater gender difference (Shaffer et al., 1997).

Male gamblers have historically constituted the majority of treatment seekers. This difference appears to be vanishing, as females begin to show higher rates of seeking and receiving treatment (Ladd & Petry, 2002b; Stinchfield & Winters, 2001). Although there are no gender differences in gambling problem severity among treatment seekers, other gender differences within this group exist (e.g., Grant & Kim, 2002; Ladd & Petry, 2002b). Treatment seeking males tend to be younger, have higher incomes, report gambling at a younger age and have been arrested for a gambling-related crime. In contrast, women tend to start gambling at an older age, progress more quickly to gambling problems, be unmarried, experience depressive symptoms, have higher credit card debt, and be in a relationship with someone with a history of addiction.

Marital Status

Those who are divorced or separated are more likely to indicate a history of gambling problems (Cunningham-Williams, Cottler, Compton, & Spitznagel, 1998). In contrast, those who are married are less likely to have symptoms of problem or pathological gambling (e.g., Volberg, 1994; Ladd & Petry 2002b). A higher proportion of treatment seekers are married (Petry & Oncken, 2002).

Ethnic Minorities

In the U.S., membership of a nonwhite ethnic minority appears to be associated with an increased risk of gambling problems (e.g., Cunningham-Williams et al., 1998; Volberg 1994; Welte et al., 2001; Wickwire, Whelan, Meyers, & Murray, 2007). In particular, African-Americans and Native Americans have been identified as at risk. This finding has been consistently supported in regional and general population studies. Shaffer and colleagues' (1997) detailed review of 120 prevalence studies included 18 studies that reported prevalence among Caucasians and at least one ethnic minority group. Each of these studies showed higher rates of problem and pathological gambling among the ethnic minority group. Similar findings have been reported in other countries (e.g., Blaszcznski, Huynh, Dumlao, & Farrell, 1998). Elevated rates of problem gambling among ethnic minorities is especially troubling because these groups appear less likely to seek treatment or call problem gambling helplines (e.g., Petry & Oncken, 2002; Stinchfield & Winters, 2001).

Problems appear more common among ethnic minorities

Socioeconomic Status

General population studies show that education and income are inversely related to level of gambling problems. In 15 studies considering this issue, participants with incomes less than US $25,000 were overrepresented among problem and pathological gamblers. In 18 studies examining educational differences, those with less than a high school degree were overrepresented among problem and pathological gamblers. Studies on treatment seeking individuals show that most had at least a high school degree (Petry & Oncken, 2002). The relation between income and treatment seeking is inconclusive.

SES is inversely related to problems

1.4 Course and Prognosis

There is no identified typical age of onset for problem and pathological gambling. The DSM-IV-TR (American Psychiatric Association, 2000) suggests the possibility of an abrupt onset of gambling problems that follows years of recreational gambling and that the onset might follow a stressor or greater exposure to gambling. While prospective studies verifying this description have not been completed, the research to date suggests that gambling problems do not necessarily grow progressively worse once symptoms appear (Hodgins & el-Guebaly, 2000; Slutske, 2006; Shaffer & Hall, 2002). For many, gambling problems often resolve without intervention (Slutske, 2006).

Onset can be abrupt after a long period without problems

It appears that people typically begin gambling during early adolescence. They usually begin wagering with family members and friends for the purpose of social interaction and entertainment (e.g., Gupta & Derevensky, 1998; Winters, Stinchfield, & Fulkerson, 1993). About a third of adolescents reported gambling before the age of 11 years and about 80% reported gambling before the age of 15 years. There is also some indication that gambling at an early age may be related to subsequent problem and pathological gambling. Adults with gambling problems tend to recall their first gambling experiences as occurring before the age of 10 years. In comparison, adult recreational gamblers remember their first gambling experiences as occurring after the age of 11 years. A minority of pathological gamblers report that their initial gambling experience occurred after the age of 19 years.

1.4.1 Negative Effects

Effects could include financial, familial, and psychological

Problem gambling can result in a wide range of negative effects. The most common consequences of problem gambling are financial. One study of 60 problem and pathological gamblers (Ladouceur, Boisvert, Pepin, Loranger, & Sylvain, 1994) revealed that 56% had spent more than $1,000 per month on gambling. Over 60% had borrowed substantial amounts of money, and 20% secured loans illegally. Over a quarter of the sample reported that they had filed for bankruptcy, and a third held considerable debt. From a different perspective, several investigators have estimated that 20% to 40% of the revenue in legal gambling venues is derived from problem and pathological gamblers (e.g., Lesieur & Rosenthal, 1998; Potenza et al., 2000).

Families of problem gamblers are often negatively affected by gamblers' activities. Lorenz and Shuttlesworth (1983) found that family members reported gambling reduced interactions within the family. Many (78%) reported thoughts of separation or divorce due to their spouses' gambling. Twelve percent of spouses indicated that they had attempted suicide. Approximately 25% of the children in these families were reported to have significant behavioral or adjustment problems, including poor school performance, drug and alcohol use, and other criminal acts. Families are also impacted financially. Sixty-five percent of spouses reported that personal savings were given to the gambler, 56% borrowed money from others to give to the gambler and 54% had been forced to borrow to meet their family's basic needs.

Gambling also affects other areas of the gambler's life. In a study of Gamblers Anonymous (GA) members (Ladouceur et al., 1994), 30% reported frequently missing work due to gambling. Theft from employers was reported by 37% and about one half of those who had stolen indicated that they had done so repeatedly, in amounts up to $5,000. Reports of other illegal acts (e.g., bad check writing, shop-lifting, etc.) were also common, as were other problems including alcohol abuse and depression (e.g., Potenza et al., 2000).

1.4.2 Natural Recovery

A substantial number of problem and pathological gamblers appear to recover from their gambling problems without professional intervention. A comparison of past year and lifetime prevalence rates suggests that at least a third of all problem and pathological gamblers successfully resolve their gambling problems (Hodgins, Wynne, & Makarchuk, 1999). A portion of those who resolved their gambling problems, possibly 10% (National Research Council, 1999; Gerstein et al., 1999), sought professional treatment. It appears that at least 20% of those who resolved their gambling problems improved without professional help (Hodgins et al., 1999; Slutske, 2006).

The majority of those who changed their gambling – with or without the help of a professional – reported that they made a conscious decision to change, rather than being forced to change by external factors. These individuals appear to be motivated by inconsistencies between their actual behavior and their preferred behavior (Hodgins, Makarchuk, el-Guebaly, & Peden, 2002). Specifically, nearly all of the individuals retrospectively reported that they ceased or changed their gambling because of financial concerns and emotional factors. A majority also reported that these motivating concerns were related to their families or children, their perception that they had hit rock bottom, and their own reflection on the advantages and disadvantages of their gambling behavior. Similar to studies on natural recovery from other addictive behaviors, most of the reasons for changing were initiated internally by the individuals and were the result of thoughtful review of how their gambling history conflicted with their personal goals and standards.

1.5 Differential Diagnosis

The presence of gambling symptoms requires differential diagnosis for at least two other disorders. The DSM-IV-TR notes that the pattern of gambling symptoms, including the borrowing of funds, lying to cover up gambling, and negative effects of gambling on daily functioning, must not be better explained by a manic episode. Second, excessive gambling and related symptoms can sometimes best be conceptualized as a component of antisocial personality disorder. In such individuals the gambling behavior might be seen as a general tendency to ignore social rules and long-range consequences.

Rule out mania and antisocial personality

1.6 Comorbidity

The literature on both general community samples as well as treatment samples suggests that problem gamblers have higher than expected rates of comorbidity with several Axis I and Axis II DSM-IV-TR disorders. The onset and pattern of these comorbid disorders is not well understood. Few studies address whether the presence or absence of other psychological problems, including substance abuse, affects problem gamblers' ability to control their gambling. Hodgins and el-Guebaly (2000) did not find that comorbid problems were differentially associated with gambling treatment or recovery. However, whether cormorbid disorders are related to gambling treatment outcome or to premature dropout from gambling treatment remains unclear.

1.6.1 Substance Use Disorders

A history of substance use disorders is commonly associated with problem gambling. In general population studies between 35% and 63% of Level 2 and 3 gamblers appear to meet criteria for at least one other substance abuse disorder

Problem gamblers often have had a substance use problem in their lifetime

at some point in their lives (Petry & Pietrzak, 2004). Rates of lifetime substance abuse disorders among nongamblers in these studies ranged from 6.5% to 19%. Gambling and lifetime alcohol problems are the most likely to co-occur. It is estimated that individuals with a gambling problem are three to five times more likely to have had an alcohol problem during their lifetime compared to recreational and nongamblers. While the base rates of both illicit drug abuse and Level 2 and 3 gambling problems are quite low, individuals with gambling problems have been found to be four to five times more likely than recreational and nongamblers to have abused illicit drugs at some time in their lives. One study of gambling and smoking found that 41% of heavy gamblers, but only 30% of recreational gamblers, were smokers (Cunningham-Williams et al., 1998).

Among treatment seeking gamblers, between 30% and 63% appear to have abused at least one substance at some point in their lives and between 5% and 39% were found to have a current substance abuse problem (Petry & Pietrzak, 2004). Alcohol is again the most common substance abused by gamblers with 26% to 63% having had alcohol problems and 4% to 23% experiencing a current alcohol problem. Gamblers in treatment have modest rates of lifetime and current illicit drug use. In contrast, the number of gamblers in treatment who smoke tobacco (between 37% and 69%) is higher than the rate of smoking among gamblers in the general community.

1.6.2 Mood Disorders

Depressive symptoms are common and likely to predate the gambling problem

Mood disorders also co-occur with gambling problems, which is not surprising as some gamble to relieve negative affect (e.g., Blaszczynski & Nower, 2002). Additionally, financial distress, an expected consequence of gambling problems, is likely to produce negative affect. Two general population studies of the relation between mood disorders and gambling problems have been published. Bland and colleagues (Bland, Newman, Orn, & Stebelsky, 1993) found that pathological gamblers, when compared to nongamblers, had significantly higher lifetime rates of depressive symptoms and dysthymia, but not major depressive disorder or bipolar disorder. Cunningham-Williams and colleagues (1998) reported that gamblers, not just those with gambling problems, were more likely than nongamblers to have experienced depression in their lifetime, including dsythymia and at least one major depressive episode. Their evidence suggested that the depressive symptoms appeared to precede gambling problems. These studies reported contradictory findings regarding whether or not those with gambling problems were more likely to experience suicidal ideation or have made a suicide attempt.

Studies of gamblers in treatment have reported elevated depressive symptoms. Rates of lifetime major depression in this population are reported to be between 33% and 76% (e.g., Specker, Carlson, Edmonson, Johnson, & Marcotte, 1996; Petry, 2005a; Winters & Kushner, 2003). Again, some evidence suggests that depressive symptoms appear to predate, and possibly contribute to, gambling problems. Evidence of bipolar disorder among those seeking treatment is inconclusive. There is strong evidence, particularly from inpatient studies, of higher than expected rates of suicidal ideation and suicide attempts among problem gamblers who seek treatment.

1.6.3 Anxiety Disorders

Cunningham-Williams and colleagues (1998) found in their general population study that Level 2 and 3 gamblers, compared to nongamblers, were more likely to experience a phobia in their lifetime, but not other anxiety disorders. Bland and colleagues (1993) reported that pathological gamblers were more likely to have experienced an anxiety disorder when compared to nongamblers, but found no differences for specific anxiety disorders. Studies of gamblers seeking treatment have noted higher levels of anxiety symptoms, but contradictory evidence about any specific anxiety disorder (e.g., Black & Moyer, 1998; Specker et al., 1996).

1.6.4 Axis II Disorders

Two published community sample studies have found significantly higher rates of antisocial personality disorder (ASPD) among those with gambling problems (Bland et al., 1993; Cunningham-Williams et al., 1998). In addition, Slutske and colleagues (2000), in a study of male veteran twins, found higher rates of ASPD in problem gamblers compared to those without gambling problems. Among studies of treatment-seeking gamblers, ASPD is frequently identified (e.g., Steel & Blaszczynski, 1998).

Few studies have considered other personality disorders. Among studies that have, modest to very high rates of personality disorder were observed in treatment-seeking gamblers. No clear conclusions can be drawn from this research.

1.7 Diagnostic Procedures and Documentation

In this section we review empirically supported diagnostic interviews and self-report measures for assessing problem gambling. Also included are measures to help monitor important treatment mediators.

1.7.1 Diagnostic Interview for Gambling Severity (DIGS)

The DIGS (Winters, Specker, & Stinchfield, 2002; Stinchfield, 2003) is a diagnostic structured interview for current or historic pathological gambling. In addition to providing an accurate and reliable diagnosis, optional DIGS questions assess gambling involvement, treatment history, mental health screening, financial difficulties, and legal problems. The DIGS was developed for use with individuals who were being clinically evaluated for possible gambling problems and is administered by a trained interviewer. It includes two questions for each of the 10 DSM-IV pathological gambling criteria and approximately five DSM-IV Axis I screening questions for each major Axis I diagnostic category. These screening questions are items selected from the Structured Clinical Interview for DSM-IV Disorders (SCID; First, Spitzer, Gibbon, & Williams, 2001) and can effectively be used to identify the need to administer

Assessment of diagnostic criteria

specific SCID modules. When used with clinical samples, the 20 diagnostic items demonstrated high internal consistency ($\alpha = .92$) as well as convergent and divergent validity (Winters et al., 2002). Factor analysis of these items revealed a unidimensional factor structure. A study with a general population found consistent psychometric support (Stinchfield, 2003). A copy of the DIGS is available from the authors at the Center for Adolescent Substance Abuse Research, Department of Psychiatry, University of Minnesota.

1.7.2 South Oaks Gambling Screen (SOGS)

Most widely used screening instrument

This 20-item self-report questionnaire is the most widely used measure for assessing problem gambling during the past year or during the respondent's lifetime (Lesieur & Blume, 1987). Scores can range from 0 to 20. Endorsing more than two items indicates problem gambling and a score greater than four indicates pathological gambling. In other psychometric studies with adult and treatment seeking samples, internal consistency was good to excellent ($\alpha = 0.86$ to 0.97), test-retest reliability was adequate ($r = 0.71$), and convergent validity was demonstrated with clinician-administered interviews ($r = 0.86$; Lesieur & Blume, 1987). The SOGS was originally cross-validated with the DSM-III diagnostic criteria. Subsequent evaluations found that the SOGS is correlated with DSM-IV diagnostic criteria for pathological gambling in both clinical and adult samples ($r = .83$ and $r = .77$, respectively) and had an overall sensitivity of 0.91 and specificity of 0.99 (Stinchfield, 2002). The SOGS has been criticized for its high false positive rate when used in prevalence studies and its overemphasis on financial problems.

1.7.3 Lie/Bet Questionnaire

The Lie/Bet Questionnaire (Johnson et al., 1977; Johnson, Hamer, & Nora, 1998) is a two item screening tool that asks if respondents have lied about how much they have gambled and whether they have felt the need to bet increasing amounts of money. These items were selected because they appeared to be the best diagnostic criteria for predicting pathological gambling. A positive response to either or both items appears to correctly differentiate Gamblers Anonymous members from recreational gamblers (Johnson et al., 1977). The measure's sensitivity is reported to be between .99 and 1.0 and its specificity between .85 and .91. No other psychometric information is available for this measure.

1.7.4 Gambling Timeline Follow-Back (G-TLFB)

Measures gambling behavior

The Timeline Follow-Back methodology is a valid and reliable strategy for assessing changes in addictive behaviors (Sobell & Sobell, 1996, 2000). The G-TLFB uses this methodology to assess recent gambling behavior over the past six months (Weinstock, Whelan, & Meyers, 2004). Individuals retrospectively fill in a calendar indicating the frequency and intensity of target behaviors. The use of memory aids (i.e., appointment books, bank and credit card statements) is encouraged in order to assist clients in remembering events or patterns. The result is a detailed record of the target behaviors that can be used to guide treatment and to monitor behavior change. Over 120 published studies have used this methodology and there are more than 35 evaluations of its psychometrics.

Information collected on the G-TLFB includes (a) type of gambling, (b) total time spent gambling, (c) amount intended to wager, (d) amount actually wagered, (e) net result of gambling, and (f) number of standard alcoholic drinks consumed. Directions for administration of the G-TLFB are provided in the toolbox of Chapter 8 (see Appendix 1). Administration begins with a trained professional providing a review of the written instructions. The instructions encourage the use of any recall strategies that might help reconstruct the previous six months of gambling. Such strategies include recording key dates directly onto the calendar (e.g., birthdays, paydays), periods of gambling abstinence or dates of gambling excursions, and patterned gambling (e.g., regular Thursday afternoon trips to the casino with friends, purchase of weekly lottery tickets). Several gambling examples are also provided to ensure that the client understands the task.

Once the measure is explained, the assessor assists the client in recording the most recent gambling episode. When the client demonstrates an ability to use the G-TLFB, he or she completes the calendar independently. The assessor should remain available in case there are questions. (For more detailed instructions on administering the Timeline Follow-Back see the 1996 manual of Sobell and Sobell). Depending on frequency of gambling behavior reported, between 20 and 40 minutes are needed to complete the G-TLFB. Initially the task may seem daunting, but once oriented to the exercise the measure becomes quite easy to complete. Most people have clear gambling patterns, even though they may not think they do. For example, major gambling events usually stand out clearly in their memories.

There is psychometric support for the G-TLFB. In a recent study, frequent gamblers completed the 6-month G-TLFB (Weinstock et al., 2004). The test-retest correlation for the six G-TLFB dimensions for the total sample and a subsample of problem gamblers ranged between .73 and .96. Fifty-eight frequent gamblers completed a convergent validity protocol. These gamblers also completed daily self-monitoring of the six G-TLFB behaviors for one month. Two-weeks following the end of the self-monitoring month, participants completed a 6-month G-TLFB. With the exception of the win/loss variable, the self-monitoring and G-TLFB data for the concurrent one-month period yielded good convergent validity (coefficients ranging from .64 to .91) for the entire sample of frequent gamblers, as well as those identified as problem gamblers. An examination of the G-TLFB win/loss data suggested that these gamblers, recreational and problem, tended to underestimate their losses in an inconsistent manner. The TLFB methodology has shown good concordance with collateral reports.

1.7.5 Addiction Severity Index – Gambling Subscale (ASI-G)

The ASI evaluates problems related to addictive behaviors and is often used to monitor changes during treatment. Sections of the scale include medi-

Provides detailed information about gambling behavior

cal history, employment, alcohol, other drug use, legal, family-social, and emotional distress. It can be administered by interview or pencil and paper. Reliability and validity is well established. The ASI-G (Petry, 2003b) is a supplement to the ASI that contains five items asking about days gambled, money spent, gambling problems experienced, distress related to gambling problems, and importance of treatment during the past 30 days. The ASI-G presented a single factor structure and internal consistency of .90. It demonstrated good temporal stability and excellent convergent validity with other measures of gambling. When combined with the ASI, this measure of gambling severity can provide helpful information about initial levels of gambling severity and changes in severity during and after treatment. The ASI-G items can be found in the 2003b paper of Petry or the book from the same author (2005a).

1.7.6 Gamblers Belief Questionnaire (GBQ)

Problem severity measure

Researchers (e.g., Ladouceur & Walker, 1996) have suggested that irrational beliefs play a causal role in problem gambling behavior, and, therefore, moderate problem gambling treatment outcome. The GBQ (Steenbergh, Meyers, May, & Whelan, 2002) is a 21-item self-report measure of gambling-related irrational beliefs. GBQ items consist of irrational statements about gambling, and respondents are asked to rate the extent of their agreement with each item using 7-point Likert scales. Test items were developed based on a review of literature and modified based on feedback from expert raters. Within a diverse sample of 403 participants, the GBQ exhibited good interitem consistency ($\alpha = .92$) and temporal reliability ($r = .77$). Factor analysis identified two factors, belief in luck/perseverance and illusion of control, that accounted for 48% of the variance. GBQ total scores were correlated with gambling behavior and measures of gambling problems. Based on these findings, the GBQ holds clear utility for aiding in comprehensive assessment of problem gambling, and developing and assessing treatment efforts.

The psychometrics of the GBQ has also been tested with a sample of problem gamblers, including some who were seeking treatment (Whelan, May, Steenbergh, Meyers, & Avondoglio, 2003). Over 30% of the participants were members of an ethnic minority group. Once again the GBQ was found to have high internal consistency ($\alpha = .85$). Consistent with a cognitive perspective on gambling, those individuals successfully completing treatment for problematic gambling evidenced a significant decrease in GBQ scores pre- to posttreatment. This scale provides a single score with higher scores reflecting greater cognitive distortion. To score, sum the ratings given to each item and then substract this sum from 147. The GBQ items are provided in the toolbox of Chapter 8 (see Appendix 2).

1.7.7 Gamblers Self-Efficacy Questionnaire (GSEQ)

The GSEQ is a 16-item self-report measure of perceived self-efficacy to control gambling behavior in a variety of high-risk situations (May, Whelan,

Steenbergh, & Meyers, 2003). Measures of self-efficacy to control addictive behaviors have been useful for monitoring behavior change, predicting maintenance of treatment gains, and identifying high-risk situations. The GSEQ was designed to efficiently monitor change in treatment and to identify clients who are at risk for relapse. For each GSEQ item respondents indicate their level of confidence in their ability to control their gambling in 16 situations. The score is the average percent confidence rating. To score the GSEQ all item scores are added and their sum is divided by 16. Higher scores are indicative of higher perceived self-efficacy. The GSEQ items are provided in the toolbox of Chapter 8 (see Appendix 3). GSEQ items were developed to represent Marlatt's (1985) categories of potential relapse situations. The GSEQ was found to have high internal consistency ($\alpha = .96$) and good test-retest reliability ($r = .86$). GSEQ scores were negatively correlated with reports of problematic gambling and individuals experiencing gambling problems scored significantly lower on the GSEQ than those who were not experiencing gambling problems. The measure also appears to have a unitary factor structure.

The GSEQ's psychometric properties have been evaluated with a sample of problem gamblers who sought treatment for gambling and problem gamblers who were not seeking treatment (Whelan et al., 2003). Over 30% of these participants were members of an ethnic minority group. The GSEQ was found to have high internal consistency ($\alpha = .97$) and appeared to measure a single factor, self-efficacy to control gambling behavior. Consistent with self-efficacy theory, those individuals who sought treatment evidenced significant increases in GSEQ scores following successful treatment. These results further supported the utility of the GSEQ with a clinical population.

Self-efficacy predictive of change and maintenance of change

2

Theories and Models

The first chapter provided an overview of problem and pathological gambling including definition, epidemiology, comorbidity, and measurement. With this information in mind, we now turn to a more conceptual focus on explanatory models of gambling problems. Clear and comprehensive theories are necessary to guide successful clinical interventions for addictive behaviors. A good theory is a useful one. Theories or models of psychopathology are judged according to their ability to produce appreciable results.

While the field of substance use disorders has several empirically based models that inform clinical interventions, the existing gambling treatment literature is not as well-established. Several models offer explanations of the etiology of problem gambling, but we believe only those with sufficient empirical support should guide case conceptualization and treatment. In this chapter we provide a review of the primary theories of problem gambling and then offer an integrated model that serves as the foundation for our Guided Self-Change treatment. The chapter concludes with an overview and rationale for this treatment model.

2.1 Gambling as an Addictive Behavior

An addictive model means that addiction research might apply to gambling

There is growing support for conceptualizing problem gambling as an addiction (e.g., Dickerson, 2003; Herscovitch, 1999; Klingemann et al., 2001; National Research Council, 1999). The essential element of addiction is that people become completely absorbed in an activity and then pursue it without regard for the negative life outcomes. Problem gambling shares characteristics and consequences with other additive behaviors, including problem drinking, tobacco use, and drug abuse (e.g., National Research Council, 1999; Wickwire et al., 2007). As noted previously, diagnostic criteria for pathological gambling reflect symptoms common to other substance use disorders. Like other addictions, problem gambling includes loss of control, preoccupation, tolerance, withdrawal, escape, cravings, and other concomitant biopsychosocial problems. There is also growing neuroscience evidence from brain imaging studies that compulsive nondrug behaviors share neurobiological commonalities with substance use disorders (Holden, 2001; Koepp et al., 1998).

These parallels between problem gambling and other addictive behaviors indicate that gambling researchers can be informed by addiction treatment literature. Being informed, in this case, does not imply the simple acceptance of alcohol or drug treatments for problem gambling. It suggests that the behavior change principles underlying treatments for these addictive behaviors are worthy of consideration in problem gambling (e.g., Herscovitch, 1999). A promising treatment program for problem gambling should embody the general principles of behavior change while also addressing elements specific to gambling. For example, it is generally accepted that irrational thinking, such as the belief in luck and the illusion of control (e.g., Ladouceur & Walker, 1996), financial issues, and the highly improbable, but still possible, pot of gold at the end of gambling's rainbow are either unique to or more prominent in gambling. These phenomena need to be addressed when using general addiction treatment principles with problem gamblers.

Table 4
Theories of Problem and Pathological Gambling

Theory	Description
Learning	• Positive reinforcement through winning and experiencing enjoyment related to gambling cause gamblers to continue to gamble. • Gambling increases due to negative reinforcement in the form of escape from unpleasant experiences, such as stress, financial worries, and difficult home situations. • Large wins serve as very powerful reinforcers. • Games that offer immediate reinforcement (e.g., slots) more readily increase gambling behavior. • Priming occurs when gambling establishments offer inducements designed to cause the gambler to resume gambling (e.g., free tokens).
Cognitive	• Individuals gamble too much because they do not understand the random nature of the gambling task or its outcome (see Table 5). • Gamblers may learn vicariously by watching others model excessive gambling or listening to others' gambling-related irrational thinking. • Problem gamblers fail to regulate their gambling behavior because they do not believe they can.
Biological	• Genetic factors may cause some individuals to have a propensity to problem gambling. • Dopamine, serotonin, and norepinephrine are thought to play a role in problem gambling due to their association with key behavioral processes. • Underactivity of dopamine in the mesolimbic reward system has been identified in problem gamblers, as well as others suffering addictive behaviors. Problem gambling and other addictions may represent efforts by individuals to compensate for this underactivity.
Disease	• An underlying disease is responsible for problem gambling. • Exposure to gambling triggers the disease process, which results in a chronic and debilitating cycle of excessive gambling and related problems. • The disease process is arrested only through complete abstinence.

Within the conceptualization of gambling as an addiction, a number of theories have been proposed to explain problem and pathological gambling. In the next few sections and in Table 4, we provide a brief overview of these theories. We conclude with a theory flexible enough to recognize the unique aspects of gambling behavior, but focused on change processes for addiction.

2.2 Learning Theories

An operant explanation of excessive gambling

Clinical scientists have widely adopted learning theories to explain gambling behavior. Early treatment approaches for problem gambling stressed the influence of operant conditioning in the acquisition and maintenance of problem gambling behavior.

Operant conditioning refers to a learning process in which the frequency or probability of a particular behavior reoccurring is influenced by the consequences that follow the behavior. Reinforcement is a key concept within this paradigm and refers to an increase in the frequency of a specific behavior due to the consequences of that behavior. Gamblers learn to associate their gambling behavior (e.g., playing slot machines) with the delivery of a reinforcer (money).

The extent to which the gambler will continue to gamble depends on various factors. The schedule on which reinforcement is delivered is one of the most important influences on behavior change. A variable ratio schedule delivers reinforcers contingent on a constantly changing number of behavioral responses. Since the respondent never knows when the next reward will occur, this schedule of reinforcement is a powerful method for producing consistent and frequent behavioral responses. In many gambling activities the frequency with which individuals are rewarded resembles a variable ratio schedule. For example, in roulette a player may win after two consecutive wagers and then lose on the next five spins. This ever-changing schedule tends to produce frequent and consistent wagering. In fact, Skinner (1953) declared that "the efficacy of such schedules in generating high rates [of response] has long been known to proprietors of gambling establishments" (p. 104).

Organisms eventually learn to discontinue a behavior when it no longer produces desirable consequences. This process of learning that a previously rewarded behavior is no longer reinforced is called extinction. Variable ratio reinforcement, on the other hand, increases resistance to extinction. Suppose a casino rigged its slot machines so that gamblers never win. Gamblers who were previously reinforced on a variable ratio schedule would have a more difficult time discriminating the change than gamblers who won, or were reinforced more frequently, and would take more time to quit playing the machines. Of course, in the real world, casinos continue to reinforce their slot machine players, which explains why problem gamblers have difficulty stopping. Even though they will lose money in the long run, the variable payout schedules condition gamblers to keep them playing.

Other behavioral concepts that warrant consideration when trying to understand gambling include the influence of large wins, immediacy of reinforcement, and priming (Petry, 2005a). A problem gambler we treated illustrates these concepts well. Yvonne had lost over $100,000 in the previous 12 months and was experiencing considerable emotional and interpersonal distress. A review of her gambling history revealed that her gambling had worsened considerably after a $60,000 win on a slot machine. Large wins are often identified as precipitants to problem gambling and some empirical evidence has supported these observations.

Yvonne preferred to play blackjack and slot machines. These are both games which offer immediate rewards that reinforce her gambling behavior. She did not engage in forms of gambling where reinforcement was delayed. Yvonne's case is prototypical, based on previous research of problem gamblers who sought treatment. Petry (2003a) reported that 63% of problem gamblers seeking treatment were slot machine or card players and only 15% primarily played the lottery. While lotteries typically yield lower numbers of problem gamblers, the growing instant win, or scratch off, lottery ticket games offer the opportunity for immediate reward. Operant theory would predict that these games have greater potential to lead to problem gambling due to the short duration between purchase and reinforcement.

Priming occurs when a reinforcer is provided noncontingently in an effort to prompt an organism to resume responding after it has stopped. Evidence that priming can be a powerful influence in initiating addictive behavior after its discontinuation is available from drug studies (Stewart & Wise, 1992). Casinos recognize the value of priming and commonly send players enticements, such as free tokens or coupons for meals or hotel rooms in the casino, which often prompt them to return to gamble. In Yvonne's case, the casino regularly sent her incentives in an effort to prime her gambling behavior. It worked. On her birthday, the casino sent Yvonne a check for $1,000 with the only stipulation that she redeem it at the casino. Unfortunately, Yvonne spent the entire $1,000 at the casino and gambled away additional money of her own.

Money is not the only reinforcer in gambling behavior. In Yvonne's case, the experience of the casino itself was a reinforcer. She loved the lights, sounds, and energy of the gaming area. The "comped" and reduced price food, beverage, hotel and resort services she received were an added incentive.

Negative reinforcement also influenced Yvonne's gambling. Negative reinforcement occurs when the removal or discontinuation of an unpleasant stimulus is contingent on a specific behavior. The addiction literature provides substantial support for the role of negative reinforcement in the maintenance of addictive behavior (Baker, Piper, McCarthy, Majeske, & Fiore, 2004). Gamblers report that they gamble for a variety of reasons, such as improving negative moods and terminating boredom (Neighbors, Lostutter, Cronce, & Larimer, 2002). In Yvonne's case, gambling helped her escape from her work and home life – areas of considerable daily stress.

Despite the reported success of behavioral interventions based on learning models for problem gambling, the great majority of gamblers do not end up gambling excessively. This is difficult to explain using an exclusively behavioral model of problem gambling. However, we believe that behavioral factors are an important component in a more comprehensive model of problem gambling.

2.3 Cognitive Theories

Erroneous thoughts lead to gambling problems

Most gamblers speak and behave in ways that reveal errors in their thinking about gambling and the factors that lead to financial success when gambling. Problem gamblers have been found to confidently endorse such thinking more often then recreational gamblers. Many of these thoughts reveal illusory correlations between their behavior and the outcomes of random events. For example, slot machine players may refuse to leave a machine that has just made a large payout. They remember occasions when continuing to play a machine after a big win resulted in a second win, or they may persist on another machine because it has not paid out in a while and assume a win is "due." This behavior can be explained by the gambler's unfounded belief that a machine is primed to pay out when it is full of money. Among lottery players, many carefully select their own numbers. They talk about lucky numbers, numbers that they saw in a dream, or numbers on a fortune cookie. The cognitive model identifies the erroneous thought processes that underlie these behaviors and postulates that these cognitive distortions are responsible for maintaining excessive gambling behavior (see Ladouceur & Walker, 1996, for a review). The slot machine player who believes that the chance of winning increases with each losing spin. This gambler is likely to persist because he or she does not want to miss the win that is believed to be just one more spin away. Such beliefs can generally be traced back to a principle cognitive error, which is the failure to recognize that randomly generated events are completely independent of one another (Ladouceur, Sylvain, Boutin, & Doucet, 2002). Table 5 provides a list of common gambling-related irrational beliefs, their descriptions, and examples.

While irrational beliefs and thought processes are common among problem and pathological gamblers, research examining gamblers' cognition during play suggests that the majority of gamblers' thoughts while gambling may be irrational – even for those who do not have a gambling problem (e.g., Coventry & Norman, 1988; Ladouceur, 2004). How does the cognitive view explain excessive gambling in some, but not in others when most gamblers think irrationally? The primary difference between nonproblem and problem gamblers appears to lie in the greater certainty with which problem gamblers hold onto their gambling-related beliefs (Ladouceur, 2004).

The cognitive perspective on problem gambling has provided a conceptual model for both information-based prevention strategies (e.g., Benshain, Taillefer, & Ladouceur, 2004; Floyd, Whelan, & Meyers, 2006; Steenbergh, Whelan, Meyers, May, & Floyd, 2004) and treatment programs designed to modify gamblers' beliefs (e.g., Ladouceur et al., 2002). However, support for the mediational role of irrational beliefs in disordered gambling has been limited. Treatment outcome studies have not examined cognitive changes from pre- to posttreatment with the exception of a single study that demonstrated decreases in irrational beliefs among gamblers treated in a multicomponent cognitive-behavioral program (Breen, Krudelbach, & Walker; 2001). The recent development of valid and reliable gambling-related cognitive measures (e.g., Raylu & Oei, 2004; Steenbergh et al., 2002) may enable future studies to explore the mechanisms of change associated with successful cognitive therapy for problem gambling.

Table 5
Common Gambling-Related Irrational Beliefs

Belief	Description	Example
Illusion of control	Overestimation of one's ability to influence the outcome of a random event.	A craps player rolls the dice softly for a low number and harder for a high number. In fact, a random event, such as the outcome of a roll of the dice, cannot be influenced by the gambler's behavior.
Gambler's fallacy	Belief that the likelihood of a specific random outcome occurring diminishes if it has occurred recently. Likewise, if a random outcome has not occurred after several trials, then it is more likely to occur in the next trial.	A roulette player sees that black has come up on the last four spins. She knows that the probability of black coming up five times in a row is very slim so she decides to wager on red for the next spin. Similarly, a lottery player may keep track of previous winning numbers in an effort to only use number combinations that have not yet won. He believes some numbers are due to win. Of course, the outcomes in these games are completely random because each spin of the roulette wheel and each lottery drawing, do not influence future outcomes. It is sometimes helpful to explain to clients that the roulette wheel has no "memory" for previous spins.
Luck	Belief that one is prone to success or good fortune. Gamblers may believe they possess an inherent tendency to win.	After winning a couple of hands of blackjack, a gambler characterizes himself as "lucky" and continues to gamble. He may explain that he is on a "lucky streak." Wins are evidence of luck and losses indicate the absence of luck. While luck may serve as a description, it does not exist empirically.
Skill orientation	Related to the illusion of control. Belief that one has certain skills or abilities that enhance one's chances of winning.	A slot player believes that experience helps him detect when a machine is "hot" or about to pay out a big win. Players may hold onto such beliefs even though they cannot influence the outcome.

Laboratory studies examining the relationship between irrational beliefs and gambling behavior have produced conflicting findings. Work in our lab by Floyd and colleagues (2006) revealed that warning messages about gambling could modify irrational beliefs and reduce the amount of money wagered. They did not demonstrate, however, that reductions in irrational beliefs caused changes in gambling behavior. Benshain and colleagues (2004) also reported reductions in erroneous gambling beliefs and gambling behavior but did not demonstrate a causal connection. Conversely, other studies (May, Whelan, Meyers, & Steenbergh, 2005; Steenbergh et al., 2004) produced modifications in irrational beliefs without concomitant changes in gambling behavior. These studies challenge the causal role that cognitive variables supposedly play in problem gambling behavior. Rather than causing problem gambling, cognitive distortions may simply be an artifact or description of behavior and have minimal explanatory value. Such a view is consistent with self-perception theory, which suggests that individuals interpret their behavior in a post hoc fashion, constructing attitudes or beliefs based on those interpretations.

Vicarious learning may also influence problem gambling. A study of Canadian high school students found elevated rates of problem gambling among students whose parents had a gambling problem, suggesting that exposure to gambling may increase children's risk of gambling problems (Gupta & Derevensky, 1998). There is evidence that psychological transmission via social learning may also be at work. Oei and Raylu (2004) studied 189 families and found positive correlations between parents' and children's scores on gambling-related cognitive distortions and problem gambling behavior. Caron and Ladouceur (2003) provided experimental evidence that exposure to those who verbalize irrational beliefs about gambling can lead to increases in gambling.

Self-efficacy is an important factor in problem gambling despite the fact that it has received relatively limited consideration in most cognitive models of disordered gambling. Perceived self-efficacy refers to one's belief in their ability to successfully engage in a specific behavior, and has a strong influence on an individual's pursuit and maintenance of behavior change. Across addictive behaviors, numerous studies have documented that self-efficacy influences whether individuals are successful in their efforts to change behavior (Bandura, 1997). May et al. (2003) provided evidence for the role of self-efficacy in problem gambling. They observed that gamblers' perceived self-efficacy levels were negatively correlated with measures of problem gambling. That is, diminishing levels of confidence to control gambling behavior were associated with increasing levels of gambling problems. Further support for the importance of self-efficacy in mediating self-regulation of gambling behavior is available from three treatment studies. Each study found that those seeking treatment for gambling problems suffered from low self-efficacy and demonstrated increases in their self-efficacy after successful treatment (Ladouceur et al., 2003; Sylvain, Ladouceur, & Boisvert, 1997; Symes & Nicki, 1997).

In summary, the cognitive perspective on gambling focuses on the role of cognitive distortions, although it is unclear whether these irrational beliefs play a causal role in problematic gambling. There is also evidence that irrational beliefs may be transmitted to others through modeling, and these beliefs have been linked to gambling behavior increases. Perceived self-efficacy has received limited attention, although both empirical evidence and clinical wisdom suggest that it is an essential component in behavior change models for problem gambling. Gamblers' cognitions are an appropriate target for intervention even if they are not directly responsible for gambling behavior. By removing gamblers' ability to explain away their behavior via irrational cognitions or increasing their confidence through planned interventions, we may ultimately enhance gamblers' self-regulation.

2.4 Biological Theories

Our understanding of the biological aspects of problem gambling has advanced over the past 15 years, and growth of research in this area suggests that our knowledge of the physiological aspects of problem gambling will continue to expand. Biological studies of problem gambling may offer unique insights into addictive processes in general (Dickerson, 2003). Unlike other substance-related addictions, gambling represents a "pure" behavioral addiction that operates independently of any foreign substances such as alcohol or cocaine. Therefore, studies examining the underlying neurochemical or neuroanatomical processes associated with gambling addiction do not have to parcel out the potential effects of the substances themselves on brain activity, a common challenge in neurobiological studies of substance use disorders (Robbins & Everitt, 1999).

Growing understanding of biological contributors

At their core, biological models link excessive gambling to dysfunctional brain activity, suggesting potential genetic bases for such dysfunction. The following sections delineate the potential genetic influences in problem gambling and explore current findings implicating neurotransmitter and neuroanatomical abnormalities in problem gambling behavior.

2.4.1 Family and Genetic Studies

Disordered gambling appears to run in families. Problem gamblers are more likely than others to report family members with gambling problems. Both family and genetic studies report increased concordance rates of problem gambling among family members. One study of veterans attending outpatient substance use and mental health clinics found that those whose parents gambled problematically were 4.7 times more likely to have a gambling problem than those whose parents did not gamble problematically (Gambino, Fitzgerald, Shaffer, Renner, & Courtnage, 1993). This study and others like it have confirmed that a family history of gambling problems is a risk factor for problem gambling. It appears that both genetic and environmental factors are responsible for this relationship.

Eisen et al. (1998) conducted a twin study that enhances our understanding of the role of genetics and environment on problem gambling. They examined the extent to which monozygotic and dizygotic twins shared symptoms of problem gambling. The rationale for such studies is that monozygotic twin pairs, who share identical genetic make up, should exhibit similar behavioral patterns if those behaviors are genetically influenced. However, because most identical twins grow up in related environments, it is impossible to know whether their behavioral similarities are due to genetics or shared experiences. By including dizygotic twins in their study, Eisen et al. were able to control for environmental influences because dizygotic twins share environments but have different genetic make up. Results from their study revealed that 35% to 54% of the variance in individual problem gambling symptoms could be explained by genetic factors.

The specific biological condition that is transmitted to affected problem gamblers is not well understood. Preliminary research has identified genetic abnormalities responsible for serotonin, dopamine, and norepinephrine receptors in problem gamblers (Comings et al., 2001). There is also evidence that the genetic vulnerability passed on by problem gamblers may place their offspring at risk for other addictive behaviors (e.g., Slutske et al., 2000).

The genetic model of problem gambling has several limitations. First, it does not explain the fact that some problem gamblers have children who never gamble excessively. Second, we would expect that identical twins would have 100% concordance since they share identical genes, yet concordance rates are much lower. Finally, a genetic model does not explain the development of gambling problems among those without a family history of problem gambling. In light of these limitations and existing research, we conclude that genetic influences are likely to be important in problem gambling, although there are several other factors that deserve consideration.

2.4.2 Neurotransmitter and Neuroanatomical Theories

Neurotransmitters have been implicated in the pathogenesis

Over the past ten years, several studies have examined the role of neurotransmitters and neuroanatomical structures in problem gambling (see Goudriaan, Oosterlaan, de Beurs, & Van den Brink, 2004). While these studies aid our understanding of the physiological basis of gambling, the complex nature of brain-behavior relationships requires considerably more research before an adequate neurobiological model of disordered gambling will emerge. Some of the most promising findings in this area, particularly those that explain the commonality between gambling and other addictive behaviors, are reviewed here.

Dopamine, serotonin, and norepinephrine, three primary neurotransmitters, have been implicated in the pathogenesis of disordered gambling behavior based on their association with key behavioral processes. Dopamine has been the most widely studied. It has been identified as a key neurotransmitter responsible for biologically mediating reinforcement processes in general and drug addiction specifically (Robbins & Everitt, 1999; Volkow, Fowler, Wang, & Swanson, 2004; Wise, 2004). Furthermore, molecular genetic studies of problem gamblers have identified abnormalities in various dopamine receptors (Goudriaan et al., 2004) and imaging studies (see below) seem to accentuate the role of dopamine in problem gambling.

Some have suggested that diminished dopamine activity in the mesolimbic reward system of some individuals may lead them to seek greater than normal levels of reinforcement through various behaviors. Gambling is one such behavior that may maintain some degree of homeostasis in dopamine activity (Blum, Cull, Braverman, & Comings, 1996). Support for this dopamine underactivity hypothesis in gamblers was provided by Reuter and colleagues (Reuter et al., 2005), who compared the mesolimbic reward system activity of pathological gamblers to normal controls during a guessing task. They used functional magnetic resonance imaging (fMRI) to study brain activity in two regions of the mesolimbic system, the ventral striatum and the ventromedial prefrontal cortex, which are responsible for reward, impulse control, and decision making, while participants tried to predict random outcomes. Pathological gamblers demonstrated reduced activity in both brain regions, which is consistent with the underactivity hypothesis. Potenza et al. (2003) found similar results, reporting reduced activity in the ventral medial prefrontal cortex of pathological gamblers during a cognitive task requiring participants to identify discrepant stimuli among a group of stimuli. It is interesting to note that individuals who have experienced damage to their ventromedial prefrontal cortex often behave like those with addictions, denying their problems and choosing immediate rewards despite negative long-term consequences (Bechara, 2003).

While theories emphasizing the role of dopamine and other neurotransmitter systems in the etiology of disordered gambling are attractive in terms of their connection to key behavioral processes, we do not yet have sufficient evidence to support their causal role. The extent to which these abnormalities precede or result from excessive gambling is unknown.

2.5 Disease Model

The disease or medical model is a well-known view of addiction. It is endorsed by 12-step programs like Gambler's Anonymous and other treatment programs, proposing that addictive behaviors result from underlying disease states within the individual. For gambling, this model suggests that exposure to gambling opportunities triggers individuals' disease, causing them to gamble in excessive and destructive ways.

The disease metaphor is a powerful one. It offers an explanation for harmful and seemingly illogical gambling, a description of the chronic course of the disease, and a solution – professional treatment and complete abstinence from gambling activities. While this view is popular within the addictions treatment community, it has limited empirical support. Research has demonstrated that many problem gamblers cycle through periods of excessive and controlled gambling (Slutske, 2006; Slutske, Jackson, & Sher, 2003). If problem gambling is due to an underlying disease state, then controlled gambling should not be possible. Yet, natural observation studies and clinical outcome data (some of which is based on the intervention we outline in Chapter 4) have demonstrated that many problem gamblers shift to controlled gambling that causes no appreciable harm. Often a shift to controlled gambling, or even abstinence, occurs without professional treatment. A recent investigation of natural recovery demonstrated that one third of untreated pathological gamblers had not experienced any gambling problems in the past year (Slutske, 2006). These data challenge the disease model and its view that gambling problems follow a chronic and worsening course. While the disease model is a popular theory that offers clients a sense of understanding, its limited empirical support should cause treatment providers to be more cautious in organizing treatment around its underlying presuppositions.

2.6 An Integrated Model of Problem Gambling

Multiple pathways to gambling problems

Independently, the behavioral, cognitive, and biological models of problem gambling are inadequate to explain the varied pathways that lead to the development of gambling problems. Problem gamblers are a heterogeneous group. Some report that both their parents had gambling problems, while others grew up in families where no one gambled. While cognitive distortions appear to play a central role for some, others seem to gamble primarily as a means to escape from difficult life circumstances. Multiple pathways may lead to similar gambling-related problems. This concept – that different events or factors may lead individuals to develop similar maladaptive behavior patterns – is referred to as equifinality and it has been demonstrated across various psychological disorders (Cicchetti, 2006).

This integrated model, which is presented in Figure 1, recognizes multiple pathways that may intersect and ultimately lead to the development of gambling problems. Those with a family history of disordered gambling may be both biologically and psychologically vulnerable to the development of gambling problems. However, without sufficient gambling experience, these individuals are unlikely to develop gambling problems. On the other hand, those without a family history of gambling problems may still experience significant gambling-related problems through a variety of other pathways. Some experience a large win, which reinforces their gambling and strengthens irrational beliefs about gambling. Others, like Ryan who is described in Chapter 5, find gambling enjoyable because of the excitement it provides or the relief it offers from stressful life experiences. A key element is that gambling begins to take on a functional role in the individual's life. As gamblers experience greater problems, their self-efficacy to control their gambling diminishes, further limiting the possibility that they will effectively self-regulate their behavior.

This integrated approach to understanding problem gambling has considerable clinical utility. While it is empirically based, it offers clinicians a flexible yet comprehensive model from which to understand and treat problem gamblers. By recognizing a variety of pathways to gambling problems, the clinician is able to relate the client's behavior to his or her unique biological, psychological, and social history. Second, the model offers a variety of potential treatment modalities (behavioral, cognitive, and psychopharmacological), which have demonstrated promising outcomes. We distinguish our model from other integrated approaches (e.g., Blaszczynski & Nower, 2002) in that the actual pathway that led to problem gambling is not necessarily directive in selecting a specific treatment modality. To date, there is limited empirical literature to guide treatment selection across psychosocial modalities, and drug therapies remain experimental. While various pathways may lead to problem gambling, psychological treatment strategies that target key cognitive and behavioral processes are likely to be effective. The Guided Self-

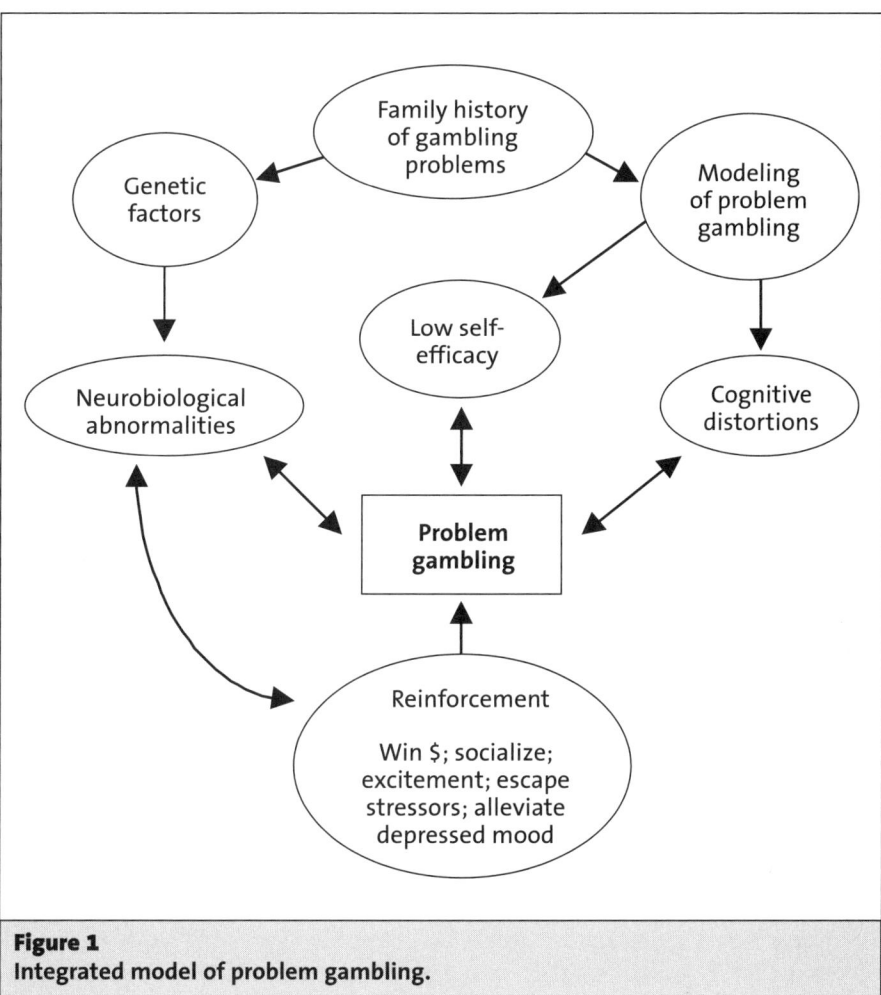

Figure 1
Integrated model of problem gambling.

Change approach addresses such processes. While this treatment approach does not include a biological component, further development and study of psychopharmacological treatments may provide future opportunity for combination therapies. The Guided Self-Change model and its rationale are briefly described in the next section.

2.7 Guided Self-Change

This integrated model for problem and pathological gambling provides a foundation for our treatment approach. The Guided Self-Change model for problem gambling, strongly influenced by the groundbreaking work of Linda and Mark Sobell on the treatment of problem drinking (Sobell & Sobell, 1993, 1998, 2005), consists of a relatively brief therapeutic intervention that relies on increasing and maintaining clients' motivation to bring their own skills and resources to bear on their dysfunctional gambling behavior. The rationale for Guided Self-Change is based on several principles that are discussed here.

A brief treatment model

2.7.1 Harm Reduction

A public health approach to addictive behavior

The use of brief, low-cost counseling is grounded in a public health perspective referred to as harm reduction. Tucker (1999) argued that our culture has a long history of individuals engaging in obsessive and repetitive behavior patterns that bring short-term rewards but eventual damage. Often we encourage and glamorize these addictive behaviors. This is clearly the case with gambling behavior that receives both corporate and state sponsorship in our society, yet can still produce social and moral stigmatization. In response to this, our society has typically adopted a zero tolerance or abstinence stance toward excessive behaviors involving alcohol, drugs, or gambling, an approach that has failed to receive consistent empirical support (Sobell & Sobell, 1993).

A harm reduction perspective requires us to develop diverse interventions and educational efforts that reach a wide range of at-risk groups through minimally intensive, low cost, but still effective programs (Curry & Kim, 1999). These interventions should be directed at reducing the harm to the individual and the community, even if the goal of abstinence is not reached. While abstinence may be the ultimate goal, the ability of the gambler to participate in gaming activities in a less harmful manner is also a desirable outcome.

Harm reduction assumes that the total elimination of harmful behavior is optimal, but difficult to achieve and maintain. This approach espouses the utility of any sustainable decrease in the damaging behavior. As it applies to addictive behavior, harm reduction treatments are pragmatic, consumer-oriented, and tolerant of alternatives to abstinence. Relaxing the abstinence requirement removes known deterrents to treatment entry and facilitates relapse prevention (Marlatt, 1998). Evidence of sustained, nonproblematic substance use following problem use has been well documented for a range of substances (e.g., Adamson & Sellman, 2001; King & Tucker, 2000), and controlled gambling has been reported among pathological gamblers who have completed treatment (Blaszczynski, McConaghy, & Frankova, 1991; Ladouceur, 2005). Indeed, programs that require abstinence typically demonstrate successful outcomes for a portion of the participants where the excessive behavior is greatly reduced but not eliminated (see Sobell & Sobell, 1993). Reductions in harmful addictive behavior have been found to meaningfully reduce the personal and social costs of the addiction.

Harm reduction, in turn, has become closely associated with the stepped care concept (Davidson, 2000; Sobel & Sobell, 2000). Stepped care consists of a set of guidelines for providing treatments sequentially according to intensity and cost. Initially, clients receive the lowest step – brief, least intrusive, and least costly treatment without compromising quality of care. More complex, intensive interventions are administered when an individual does not respond to a less intensive step. Variations of the Guided Self-Change treatment described below can be used as the initial or early step when treating alcohol problems (Sobell & Sobell, 2000).

2.7.2 Rapid Change Response

There is a growing recognition that a significant amount of therapeutic change often occurs within the first few treatment sessions (Wilson, 1999). This rapid change response, as it has been called, predicts both the eventual outcome of treatment and the maintenance of treatment change. The association between early treatment change and eventual outcome has been found with a variety of presenting problems (Wilson, 1999), and the rapid treatment response has been noted in treatments for various addictions (Miller, 2000; Sobell, Breslin, & Sobell, 1998). It has also kindled an interest in the potential value of brief treatments that ignite change within just a few sessions. Research has demonstrated more therapy is not necessarily better and brief interventions can motivate sustainable changes. Various characteristics of cognitive behavioral treatments have been linked to rapid change, including clinical treatment guidelines, assessment that is linked to treatment, interventions that begin early in treatment, and periodic review of treatment goals (McGinn & Sanderson, 2001). Recent research has supported the effectiveness of brief treatment of gambling problems (Hodgins, Curry, & el-Guebaly, 2001; Lipinski, Whelan, & Meyers, in press; Petry et al., 2006).

How can brief treatment and rapid change create sustainable change in an individual with a severe addiction? For many who present with addictive behavior problems, brief interventions may be sufficient to motivate clients to learn a general strategy for identifying and responding to high-risk situations. Brief treatments can also encourage the natural recovery processes discussed in Chapter 1 and help clients utilize their own natural resources to maintain change. This perspective has been supported in studies that have found that brief interventions, between two and eight sessions, significantly reduce the harm associated with addictive behaviors.

Sobell and Sobell (1998) have proposed that the therapeutic value of short-term, harm reduction treatments might be enhanced by the inclusion of four treatment components.

1. Increase individuals' motivation to avoid or control the problem behavior by identifying the adverse consequences of such behavior and by having participants join with the therapist to determine their own treatment goals.
2. Help individuals identify situations that pose a risk of engaging in the addictive behavior and use alternative ways of dealing with those situations.
3. Help individuals recognize their strengths for dealing with high-risk situations.
4. Help individuals develop plans for implementing personal strategies to manage high-risk situations.

2.7.3 Self-Change

Consistent with Bandura's (1977) social cognitive theory, the Guided Self-Change approach is intended to facilitate self-change by having clients play a central role in determining and enacting plans for change. One way to facilitate this self-determined change process is to encourage the individual to set their own treatment goal rather than have one imposed by the therapist. This goal may be abstinence or continuing the behavior in a more controlled fashion. Further self-determination is derived from allowing the person to thoughtfully

Treatment can be informed by natural patterns of change

revise the goal as the treatment progresses. From a motivational perspective, the major concern is not the type of goal a client will pursue, but rather how that decision is made. Bandura argued that people perform better when they have actively selected their goals than when their goals have been designated by others. Goal attainment, in turn, is important for enhancing self-efficacy, which is positively related to outcome.

The potential benefits of treatment seekers selecting their own goals seem to greatly outweigh the efficiencies when the treatment provider decides on the goal. Provider-imposed goals may also create resistance and barriers to change. Furthermore, there is evidence that individuals seeking treatment prefer to have a choice.

2.7.4 Motivational Approach

Motivation is dynamic and can be influenced

Miller and Rollnick (2002) argued that the act of increasing one's commitment to change can be sufficient for many individuals to make meaningful inroads into problematic behavior. Another basic assumption of Guided Self-Change is that this motivation to change is a dynamic state open to influence by a therapist or others. Ambivalence about the target behavior is normal, constitutes an important obstacle to recovery, and can be resolved through a flexible alliance between client and therapist.

Motivational interviewing style is a directive and client-centered counseling style that is designed to enhance motivation for change in addictive behaviors. It blends principles drawn from motivational psychology, client centered therapy, and the processes of change in natural recovery from addiction (Prochaska & DiClemente, 1986; Prochaska, DiClemente, & Norcross, 1992). Positive results have been identified in several interventions conducted from this perspective. Despite the apparent complex blend of therapeutic elements in motivational interviewing, the therapist's skills and strategies have been well established and detailed training modules are available in the literature (Miller & Rollnick, 2002; Miller et al., 1992).

The integrated model of problem gambling that we outlined in this chapter borrows from several valuable theoretical models and provides a foundation for the application of Guided Self-Change treatment for problem gamblers. In the next chapter we discuss diagnostic and assessment issues related to problem gambling and describe treatment options.

3

Diagnosis and Treatment Indications

In this chapter we review diagnostic decisions, assessment issues, and treatment alternatives for problem gambling. We describe the ideal and the most efficient methods for identifying problem and pathological gambling. Next, we discuss other assessment domains that are either essential or helpful in the delivery of the Guided Self-Change for Gambling (GSCG) treatment. The final section provides an overview of other treatment options that have some empirical support.

3.1 Diagnostic Assessment

No "gold standard" currently exists to determine the presence of pathological gambling. Without absolute criteria, diagnostic interviews have become the accepted assessment strategy. The DIGS, described in Chapter 1, is the best supported diagnostic interview for pathological gambling. The DIGS includes 20 items, two for each DSM-IV-TR diagnostic criterion. If a person answers affirmatively to either or both of the questions for any one diagnostic criterion, then he or she meets that specific criterion. Other DIGS items, as detailed in Chapter 1, can be used to collect additional clinical information, but administration is optional. As a result, a reliable and valid diagnosis can be secured within five to ten minutes. There is psychometric support for using the 20 gambling-related diagnostic questions alone.

No gold standard

An alternative to the diagnostic interview is a self-administered screening measure. Several such measures are available. The past-year SOGS, also described in Chapter 1, is brief and is the most widely used, psychometrically evaluated self-report measure in the literature. Scores of 3 or 4 on the SOGS indicate problem gambling. Scores greater than four indicate pathological gambling. It is well accepted that standard SOGS cutoff scores identify some nonpathological gamblers as pathological gamblers and the measure overemphasizes financial issues.

3.2 Treatment Indications

The gambling treatment literature does not support that differences in the intensity of gambling problems or the type or pattern of gambling require different treatment approaches. A determination of whether an individual meets

Concern about gambling and its harm justifies treatment

diagnostic criteria for pathological gambling is helpful, but not essential when making a decision to use GSCG. Concern about an individual's gambling and its related harm justifies treatment. These concerns may include the gambler's judgment that gambling is harmful to one's self or to significant others, or that family members, friends, a member of the clergy, coworkers, etc., are concerned about the gambling.

While the criteria we use to determine whether an individual is likely to benefit from GSCG is fairly straightforward, there are several contraindications that should be considered in ruling out the application of this treatment. If a person presents with suicidal ideation or other emergent psychological crises, then Guided Self-Change treatment should not be pursued. As discussed in Chapter 1, those who seek gambling treatment have higher than expected rates of suicide and suicidal thinking. It is essential that this domain be assessed. For those who are in immediate crisis, a referral for appropriate intervention to resolve the threat should be initiated and GSCG may be pursued once the client is stable.

Clients who present with complicated comorbid disorders are also poor candidates for GSCG. These include individuals who are psychotic or abusing multiple substances. In such cases, treatment should first target the most severe psychological symptoms. Gambling treatment may be offered once an adequate level of psychosocial functioning has been achieved.

For problem gamblers who have common comorbid disorders, such as depression or single substance abuse, GSCG treatment may be pursued. As discussed in Chapter 1, rates of depression are high among those with gambling problems. GSCG treatment may aid in reducing depression levels by positively impacting gambling behavior, which improves other areas of the gambler's life. In cases where comorbid issues are present, such as depression or marital problems, we usually try to understand gambling in relation to these problems; however, we do not expect that successful gambling-focused treatment will solve them. Referral to other providers to specifically address such issues is helpful.

Alcohol problems are also common among those who seek treatment for gambling. Our experience is that the Guided Self-Change treatment, which was initially developed to address problem drinking, can be successfully used to simultaneously address both gambling and drinking problems (Lipinski, Whelan, & Meyers, in press). We describe the assessment of substance-related issues in the next section.

3.3 Clinical Assessment

Our general approach to assessment is to efficiently assess variables that have implications for the delivery of the GSCG treatment. In addition to assessing gambling behavior, we encourage clinicians to examine potential treatment mediators, systemic factors, and comorbid psychopathology. There is no substitute for a thorough assessment of these domains. Once evaluated, these factors can be understood in relation to the integrated model of problem gambling and the Guided Self-Change philosophy presented in Chapter 2. To illustrate the clinical assessment and case conceptualization process, we will discuss

Yvonne, the airline pilot whose case we briefly described in the learning theory section of Chapter 2.

3.3.1 Gambling Behavior

A clear picture of a client's gambling is essential for GSCG treatment to be successful. We have found that an understanding of the type and pattern of gambling, its intensity, the amount the gambler intends to risk and actually risks, and the financial costs of gambling are most helpful. The Gambling Timeline Follow-Back (G-TLFB) is an efficient method for gathering this data.

Gambling Timeline Follow-Back provided details about this behavior

To illustrate the utility of G-TLFB data, we return to the case of Yvonne, who completed a 6-month version of the G-TLFB at the outset of treatment. Over the previous six months, Yvonne reported gambling on approximately 20% of the days for a total of 456 hours. She lost about $25,300 during this period (this does not include the $60,000 she had won and then lost approximately 12 months prior to treatment). Her heaviest gambling days occurred on weekday evenings. On days she gambled, she typically planned to wager between $400 and $500 and would gamble up to 12 hours. She exceeded this planned limit about half the time. Gambling excursions following a sizable win regularly resulted in excessive gambling. Yvonne's drinking varied across episodes, but never exceeded four standard drinks. The presence or absence of alcohol consumption appeared to have no relationship to her gambling. While reviewing the G-TLFB data with Yvonne she described situations when she maintained or failed to maintain her limits. It became clear that her gambling was heaviest during times of family stress. Her gambling allowed her to escape the negative affect she experienced when interacting with her family.

As we describe in Chapter 4, the assessment process can be therapeutic in the sense that it helps clients better understand their gambling behavior and often motivates them for change. As Yvonne examined her cumulative losses over the 6-month period, as well as the amount of time she had spent gambling, she expressed a growing desire for change. In summary, the G-TLFB method informs the delivery of GSCG treatment in three ways. First, as clients' examine their gambling over a 6-month period it allows them to better understand whether their gambling involvement is consistent with their values and goals. Second, discussion of G-TLFB data often prompts clients to begin talking more concretely about what specific behavioral changes they desire. Third, it offers clients an opportunity to discuss particular gambling situations that, in turn, guide the functional analysis and problem-solving components of the GSCG treatment. In Yvonne's case, it became clear that gambling helped her escape from stressful family interactions. Treatment could then address these situations specifically using problem-solving strategies developed from a functional analysis of her gambling behavior.

3.3.2 Assessment of Possible Treatment Mediators

Three variables that may mediate treatment outcome should be evaluated: gambling-related cognitive distortions, self-efficacy to control gambling, and

Assess mediators of treatment outcome

readiness for change. While the GSCG treatment is not designed to target these variables directly, its application should be tailored to fit the unique presentation of the client in relation to these potential mediators.

As described in our integrated model in Chapter 2, irrational thought processes related to gambling may contribute to the maintenance of problem gambling. To assess clients' cognitive distortions, we use the Gamblers Beliefs Questionnaire (GBQ; see Chapter 1 and Appendix 2), which provides an index of gamblers' irrational beliefs. For clients whose GBQ scores are elevated (means and confidence intervals for clinical and general population samples appear in Table 6) and whose verbal reports evidence strong cognitive distortions, treatment may require a cognitive modification component. Ladouceur et al. (2002) provided a thorough description of the cognitive modification process, which can be integrated within the GSCG treatment. In our initial assessment, Yvonne's GBQ scores were not significantly elevated and her discussions in session made it clear that she generally understood the independence of random events and seemed to hold no significant irrational beliefs about gambling. For clients who hold strong irrational beliefs, individual GBQ items can be used within Phase 3 to address specific beliefs that serve as antecedents of gambling episodes.

Our integrated model identified self-efficacy as another key variable. To assess gamblers' perceptions of their ability to control gambling, we use the Gambling Self-Efficacy Questionnaire (GSEQ; see Chapter 1 and Appendix 3). Many problem gamblers present for treatment with low GSEQ scores (means and confidence intervals for clinical and general population samples

Table 6
Means and Standard Deviations for GBQ and GSEQ

Measure	Statistics	Clinical Sample[1]	Nonclinical Sample[2]		
		Pathological Gamblers	Nonproblem Gamblers	Problem Gamblers	Pathological Gamblers
GBQ	Mean	68.3	52.5	60.7	70.9
	SD	21.4	22.2	18.8	21.5
	95% CI[3]	± 20.1	± 20.8	± 17.6	± 20.2
	n	117	317	22	32
GSEQ	Mean	49.1	93.2	71.4[4]	
	SD	29.3	12.0	24.3	
	95% CI	± 21.4	± 8.8	± 17.8	
	n	117	253	56	

[1] Data are from Whelan et al. (2003) sample of pathological gamblers seeking treatment.
[2] Data for the Nonclinical GBQ sample are from Steenbergh et al. (2002) and the Nonclinical GSEQ data are from May et al. (2003). Both studies used the South Oaks Gambling Screen to classify individuals.
[3] 95% Confidence Interval.
[4] The May et al. (2003) study combined data for problem and pathological gamblers.

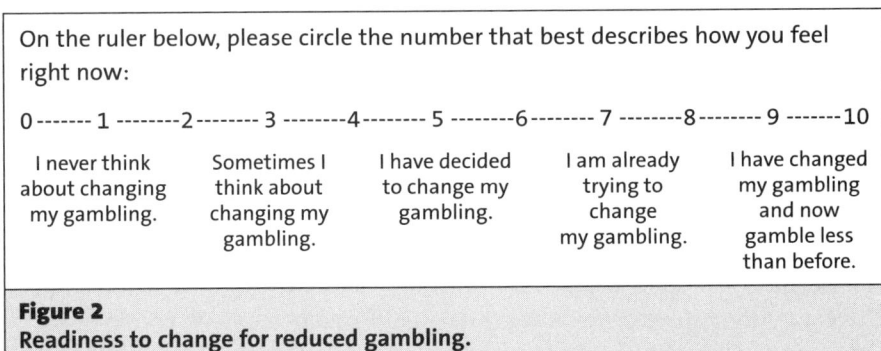

Figure 2
Readiness to change for reduced gambling.

appear in Table 6). However, for those who report low self-efficacy in specific situations, the clinician should carefully monitor the client's confidence to manage gambling and subsequent behavior in those situations and tailor treatment to address them. For example, Yvonne reported moderate levels of self-efficacy to control her gambling except when she was angry or when there were fights at home. In those situations she rated her self-efficacy to control her gambling at 10%, meaning that she thought there was only a 10% chance she could regulate her gambling under those conditions. Treatment should focus on improving the client's ability to manage these high-risk events and, consequently, increasing her self-efficacy for controlling future challenges.

The transtheoretical model of change (Prochaska, DiClemente, & Norcross, 1992) suggests that individuals change addictive behaviors by working through five stages – precontemplation, contemplation, preparation, action, and maintenance. We have found this model helpful in our work with problem gamblers. Depending on the client's stage of change, the clinician might initially pursue different session objectives. For example, problem gamblers in the precontemplation stage should be encouraged to consider the consequences of their gambling behavior with the hope of moving them onto the contemplation and preparation stages. The University of Rhode Island Change Assessment adapted for gambling (URICA-Gambling; Petry, 2005b) has demonstrated validity in identifying stages of change with problem gamblers. An alternative is the stages of change ruler, which is a one-item measure that has been found to be highly correlated with longer questionnaires (LaBrie, Quinlan, Schiffman, & Earleywine, 2005). The advantage of the change ruler is that it is simple and brief. A copy of the change ruler we use with gamblers appears in Figure 2. Our assessment of Yvonne suggested that she was in the contemplation stage. While problem gamblers may present for treatment at different stages of change, the motivational interviewing approach described in the next chapter focuses on moving gamblers along the behavior change continuum.

3.3.3 Systemic Factors

The context within which the gambler lives may influence the delivery of treatment. Contextual variables, including relationships, financial issues, and legal problems deepen the clinician's understanding of individual cases of problem gambling. Understanding the nature and quality of relationships the gambler has with significant others and family members is essential. For some gamblers, like Yvonne, relationship turmoil is an ongoing stressor that contributes to their inclination to gamble. For others, their gambling problems appear to precede and cause their relationship problems. Regardless of the temporal sequence, relationship difficulties and gambling problems often become part of an escalating cycle of destruction. Growing financial problems due to excessive gambling cause those close to the gambler to become increasingly distraught. As the gambler's closest relationships become strained, gambling can become a refuge, which further exacerbates existing problems. A basic clinical interview can provide some data on the gambler's perception of his or her relationships. However, we often find that relationship satisfaction assessment can be especially helpful. The dyadic adjustment scale (Spanier, 1976) is a commonly used measure of this variable.

One of the interesting aspects of Yvonne's case was that her spouse also gambled frequently. In fact, on some occasions he also spent more than he had intended, although his gambling was not nearly as problematic as Yvonne's. An interview with him helped us better understand his role in Yvonne's gambling. We were surprised to find that both he and Yvonne identified gambling as the only activity that they enjoyed together.

Financial devastation is a hallmark of problem gambling. Even Yvonne, who earned over $100,000 per year, began to suffer the financial consequences of her addiction. She had begun to use what she called "creative financing" to support her gambling addiction. She borrowed from her retirement account and transferred credit card balances. Her husband did not manage their finances so he was unaware of Yvonne's use of family funds for gambling. While the G-TLFB can provide a valid presentation of the client's gambling, research suggests that gamblers tend to underreport their gambling behavior. It is often helpful to have clients compile a list of all existing debts and all sources of income to get a better sense of their financial health.

Finally, it is important to consider legal issues that may complicate a client's recovery. Some clients commit illegal acts to acquire gambling money. Those who are caught and prosecuted are sometimes required to seek treatment. While legal problems may serve as a significant motivator for some clients, others may be less committed to treatment. Identifying the latter group is difficult. However, those who have a history of antisocial behavior may be particularly difficult to treat.

3.3.4 Comorbid Psychopathology

Given their high rates of comorbidity with problem gambling, the presence of substance use and mood disorders should be evaluated in the assessment phase. We typically use the clinical interview to gather information in these areas, but assessment instruments may also be used. Those who demonstrate clinically significant substance use or mood disorders should be referred for psychotherapy or pharmacological interventions.

We regularly screen for alcohol problems using the Alcohol Use Disorders Identification Test, or AUDIT (Saunders, Aasland, Babor, De La Fuente, & Grant, 1993). This 10-item self-report measure has considerable psychometric support. Total scores of eight or above identify individuals who may be at risk for, or who have experienced alcohol problems during the past year. Clients who evidence alcohol problems may be treated concurrently with the GSCG treatment. In such cases, the GSCG treatment can be modified so that the treatment principles are applied to the client's gambling and drinking problems.

3.4 Treatments

We draw three conclusions from gambling treatment literature. First, problem and pathological gamblers effectively respond to treatment. In particular, cognitive-behavioral treatments (CBT) have shown clear promise for modifying problem gambling (e.g., National Research Council, 1999; Toneatto & Millar, 2004). A recent meta-analysis of 22 studies of psychological interventions for problem gambling reported an average effect size of 2.01 at posttreatment and 1.59 after an average follow-up of 17 months (Palleson, Mitsem, Kvale, Johnsen, & Molde, 2005). Second, when compared to the treatment of other addictive behaviors, problem gambling interventions have only begun to undergo rigorous empirical evaluation. Many reports of problem gambling treatments are limited to case studies and uncontrolled treatment evaluations. Third, little work has been done to develop brief treatments designed to address problem gambling. Brief outpatient treatments have been successful with other addictive behaviors, but have received limited attention as treatments for problem gambling. In this section we briefly review alternative or adjunctive treatments to GSCG.

Other treatment with empirical support

Contemporary treatment models have recognized the value of combining behavioral and cognitive components, which offer a more comprehensive view of problem gambling and its treatment. Ladouceur and his colleagues developed what has become perhaps the most widely studied and supported CBT for gambling problems. Ladouceur and colleagues' (2002) treatment approach includes five primary components: educational efforts designed to teach gamblers about games of chance; correcting cognitive distortions; problem-solving skills training; social skills training; and relapse prevention. The treatment is delivered in an average of 17 one-hour sessions and those who completed treatment, when compared to those who were not in treatment, realized significant improvement. Ladouceur's program has demonstrated effectiveness for both adolescent and adult problem gamblers in individual therapy. A group treatment based on this model also reduced problem gambling among adults (Ladouceur et al., 2003).

Petry et al. (2006) developed and tested an eight-session CBT package. It is more behavioral than Ladouceur's treatment, although it does incorporate a cognitive modification component. Other treatment strategies include a functional analysis of gambling behavior, identification of gambling triggers and new methods to address them, development of alternative leisure activities, reinforcement of nongambling activities, helping the client deal with cravings and urges, managing interpersonal conflict, and making decisions with a longer term perspective. GA attendance is also encouraged. Results from a clinical trial of this treatment suggest that it is efficacious (Petry et al., 2006). Relative to GA referral or a client-directed workbook condition, this CBT package produced superior results at 12-month follow-up. Those who received the CBT package reduced their gambling from 13.3 days per month to 6.0 and their monthly gambling expenditure dropped from $1,260 in the month prior to therapy to only $76 at the 12-month follow-up.

One of the interesting findings noted in the aforementioned study was the relative effectiveness of GA and workbook only conditions. Both conditions produced significant reductions in monthly gambling expenditures and days gambling. These data are consistent with others indicating that GA and self-help programs can significantly curtail problem gambling. For those clients who are unable to receive individual therapist-guided treatment, GA or other self-help programs may be effective. The Petry et al. (2006) study suggested that GA attendance provided additional benefit to those in the CBT condition. GA is particularly attractive for some because of its structure and availability. It offers gamblers an atmosphere of acceptance, a social support system, and structured guidelines for behavior change. GA meetings are often available within a short drive for most gamblers, and larger cities offer multiple meetings throughout the week.

Self-directed treatment manuals, or bibliotherapies, are a minimally intensive and potentially effective treatment alternative for problem gamblers. While they appear to be less effective than therapist-delivered CBTs, they fill an important niche in a stepped care treatment approach. In addition to the Petry self-help manual mentioned previously, two others have been developed and tested. Dickerson, Hinchy, and England's (1990) self-help workbook included education about gambling problems, self-monitoring, functional analysis, goal setting, and relapse prevention. A similar workbook developed by Hodgins and el-Guebaly (2000) included information on a cognitive-behavioral model of problem gambling, relapse prevention, and natural recovery. A combination of a single motivational interview and this self-help manual produced significantly greater reductions in problem gambling than the manual alone (Hodgins et al., 2001).

Pharmacological interventions for problem gambling are based on the biological model of problem gambling that we discussed in Chapter 2. Three drug classes have been studied in work with problem gamblers: serotonin reuptake inhibitors (e.g., Grant et al., 2003), opioid antagonists (e.g., Grant et al., 2006), and mood stabilizers (e.g., Pallanti et al., 2002). Existing pharmacotherapy research is in its early stages, largely focused on establishing the efficacy of these treatments. The research that is available provides little direction for treating clinicians due to several limitations. First, most studies have included single cases or small samples without adequate controls. Second, outcomes have generally been evaluated in terms of global clinical ratings or other measures with limited psychometric support. Third, long-term follow-up assessment has not been conducted. At this point pharmacotherapy for problem gambling is largely experimental. Presently there are no FDA-approved pharmacotherapies for problem gambling. Future treatments for problem gambling may include combined psychological and pharmacological interventions, as these have proven effective in other addictive behaviors.

4

Treatment

In this chapter we present the practice guidelines for Guided Self-Change for Gambling, which we also refer to as GSCG. These guidelines provide you with a sequential set of objectives, and the steps and tools needed to reach these objectives. The treatment's five phases described below can be delivered in five sessions, but for some clients completing all phases may require additional sessions. Attendance and treatment compliance are important, but as the clinician, you need to consider adapting the pace and scheduling of treatment to fit the client's progress through the phases. The same flexibility is needed for treatment content. There are core components that must be included in each phase of the treatment process, but individual sessions can, and should be, tailored to each client's needs. Use the motivational interviewing style to prompt the client to move through the phases. We direct rather than dictate the content of each session.

Description of Guided Self-Change for Gambling

4.1 Method of Treatment

The objectives of GSCG are as follows. (a) Complete a careful and detailed examination of the client's gambling behavior. (b) Make a choice about change and the related treatment goal. (c) Learn about the triggers and consequences of the client's gambling. (d) Learn to control the antecedents of gambling and implement alternative behaviors. (e) Learn to successfully maintain changes in gambling.

It is important throughout treatment to maintain a motivational interviewing style. Homework assignments are used to reinforce the focus of each treatment phase, and to promote thinking about the next step in the process. Before describing the five treatment phases, let us briefly describe some basic principles of this treatment approach.

4.1.1 Basic Principles

Setting the Stage for Change
Motivation for change is often facilitated when individuals identify a discrepancy between their current pattern of behavior and their perceived ideal behavior. Based on this perspective, commitment to change may be enhanced by strategies that help identify such discrepancies. For example, personalized feedback of assessment results can be persuasive input for convincing clients of the harmful and atypical aspects of their past behavior and of the negative ramifications of continuing this behavior.

Motivational self-management approach

The assessment process not only produces data about the client but also serves as the initial step in the therapeutic process. This will very likely be the first time that clients have thought seriously about their gambling, the amount of money they expend, and problems or distress related to gambling. Many successful brief interventions include such client feedback. This process, referred to as a "running start" assessment, can be extremely important in setting the stage for change by allowing clients to begin to evaluate their current patterns of behavior by contrasting those patterns with their ideal behaviors.

Identifying the Goal of Change

Self-change is facilitated when the client takes responsibility for his or her behavior and goals. This is promoted early in treatment by having the client determine the treatment goal. In every subsequent session, you will have the client reconsider the goal and the client's self-efficacy for achieving that goal. Based on information from the assessment and subsequent feedback, the client is encouraged to set a treatment goal of abstinence or of continuing the behavior in a more controlled fashion. From the perspective of motivation to change, the major concern is not the type of goal a client will pursue, but rather how that decision is made. People perform better when they actively select their goals rather than when their goals are provided by a therapist.

Implementing the Change

A functional analysis of problem behavior and the modification of this behavior to more adaptive alternatives are common components of behaviorally-oriented interventions. The therapeutic value of this treatment is enhanced by helping clients learn how to (a) identify specific situations that put them at risk for engaging in the problem behavior, and (b) use their personal strengths and resources to develop alternative behaviors for dealing with these situations. This process allows clients to enhance existing skills as well as to develop new skills for implementing behavior change.

Maintaining the Change

A goal of any treatment targeting behavior change is to maintain treatment gains over time. To this end, successful brief interventions have targeted relapse prevention and its two major components. The first is the identification of situations in which the client might be at a high risk for relapse, and the development of plans for dealing with those situations. The second component focuses on the cognitive aspects of relapse. Clients are encouraged to adopt the perspective that relapses may occur, and that although a lapse is unfortunate, the way in which the relapse is conceptualized and responded to is more important. Clients are informed that relapses should (a) be interrupted as soon as possible to minimize negative consequences, (b) be considered as learning experiences that identify unrecognized high-risk situations or inadequate coping methods, and (c) not be attributed to personal failings but rather to situational factors that can be dealt with successfully in the future.

Motivational Interviewing Style

As described in Chapter 2, this treatment approach assumes that motivation is a dynamic state that we can and should influence. The therapist's style of interacting must be both directive and client-centered. It blends concepts and strategies from diverse areas of psychology to enhance clients' motivation to change their excessive behavior.

The motivational style attempts to elicit behavior change by helping clients explore and resolve their ambivalence about the addictive behavior. Our responsibility is to engage the client in a partnership for change. Reflective listening is employed to minimize resistance to intervention and change. Arguments and direct confrontation are avoided, "rolling with resistance" rather than directly opposing it. A primary goal of this style is to support client self-efficacy and optimism by targeting client competencies and strengths. We strongly encourage anyone unfamiliar with this approach to read Miller and Rollnick's "Motivational interviewing: Preparing people to change addictive behavior" (2002), and/or attend a motivational interviewing workshop. Another helpful resource is a free motivational intervention manual available from the Substance Abuse and Mental Health Service Administration (2000). Information about this manual is included in Chapter 6.

Clinical Pearl
An Overview of Motivational Interviewing Style

The challenge for the therapist is to approach each phase of the treatment in such a way that the client can experience success before moving on to the next phase. Adopting a motivational interviewing approach to treatment can facilitate this movement. The material presented here provides a brief synopsis of motivational interviewing.

What is motivational interviewing?
- Motivational interviewing is a directive but client-centered counseling style.
- It elicits behavior change by helping clients explore and resolve ambivalence.
- It helps to resolve ambivalence by increasing discrepancy between the client's current behavior and desired goals while minimizing resistance.
- During motivational interviewing empathic listening is essential to minimize resistance.

How do motivational techniques help people change?
- By recognizing their high-risk behavior through personalized feedback on previous gambling behavior.
- Using decisional balance exercises, goal statements, and self-evaluation to judge how serious a problem their gambling is for them in relation to other life issues.
- Looking at ways to begin the process of change by identifying strengths and developing action plans.

The basics of motivational interviewing:
- Express empathy through reflective listening.
- Develop discrepancy between client's goals or values and current behavior.
- Avoid arguments and direct confrontation.
- Roll with resistance rather than opposing it directly.
- Support self-efficacy and optimism.

> **Clinical Pearl**
> **Statements to Avoid**
>
> Below we list ways of responding that indicate that a therapist is not listening reflectively. Rather than create an environment of confidence and trust, the therapist establishes roadblocks that impede the therapeutic relationship and potentially increase resistance to change.
>
> - **Ordering or directing.** Direction is given with the voice of authority.
>   - *You really need to stop that.*
>
> - **Warning or threatening.** An overt or covert threat of impending negative consequences if the advice or direction is not followed.
>   - *Continuing down this path will certainly lead you into further trouble.*
>
> - **Giving advice, making suggestions, or providing solutions.** A recommended course of action based on the clinician's knowledge and personal experience.
>   - *Have you tried ...?*
>
> - **Persuading with logic, arguing, or lecturing.** The assumption of such messages is that the client has not reasoned through the problem adequately and needs help to do so.
>   - *The facts are that ...*
>
> - **Moralizing, preaching, or telling clients their duty.** Statements that contain such words as "should" or "ought" to convey moral instructions.
>   - *You should ...*
>
> - **Judging, criticizing, disagreeing, or blaming.** These messages imply that something is wrong with the client or with what the client has said.
>   - *I don't think you are right.*
>
> - **Agreeing, approving, or praising.** Unsolicited approval can interrupt the communication.
>   - *I think that you are absolutely right.*
>
> - **Humiliating, ridiculing, or labeling.** Overt disapproval and intent to correct a specific behavior or attitude.
>   - *How could you do that?*
>
> - **Interpreting or analyzing.** Therapists are frequently and easily tempted to impose their own interpretations on a client's statement and to find some hidden, analytical meaning.
>   - *I don't believe you really mean that.*
>
> - **Reassuring, sympathizing, or consoling.** Therapists often want to make the client feel better by offering consolation.
>   - *I'm sure everything will be fine.*
>
> - **Questioning or probing.** In fact, insensitive questioning can interfere with the spontaneous flow of communication and divert it in directions of interest to the therapist instead of the client.
>   - *Why?*
>
> - **Withdrawing, distracting, humoring, or changing the subject.** Distraction strategies can divert communication and imply that the client's comments are unimportant.
>   - *Let's talk about that later.*

4.1.2   Phase 1: Running Start Assessment

The primary goals of this phase are to obtain information regarding the client and his or her gambling behavior, and develop the client's motivation to change. This phase should be viewed as much more than an information-gathering opportunity. We must also engage the client in the treatment and enhance the client's motivation for change. During this initial phase you should strive to develop a positive relationship with the client. Adopting a motivational, empathic style of interaction as described in the previous section can facilitate this. Although this style should be used throughout treatment, it is particularly important in early interactions that lay the foundation for the therapeutic relationship.

Enhance motivation to change

As we previously described, the assessment process is an integral part of the motivational effort and the treatment process. Often, when an individual receives treatment for their gambling behavior, it is the first time they have seriously considered the amount of money and time that they have spent gambling, and the corresponding negative consequences. A thorough understanding and consideration of these consequences can serve as valuable motivators for behavior change.

Assess gambling behavior

Components of Phase 1

Promote the client's engagement in treatment. People arrive for treatment for different reasons. Some come because of a recent gambling episode, others because gambling has resulted in problems at work or at home. Not infrequently, a person shows up because of the demands of a spouse, friend, a member of the clergy, or even a child. A few arrive for treatment because of pending legal problems or as a mandate from an employer. We begin the first session by listening to clients' stories and the reasons they are here. Ask the question, "What can I do for you?" Using a motivational interviewing style will help build a connection with the client and facilitate their consideration of change. It is crucial during this session to maintain a nonjudgmental view of their gambling.

Briefly explain the treatment. Provide clients with information regarding the expected length of treatment, treatment expectations, treatment components, and the importance of completing homework assignments. We find it helpful to emphasize the clients' role in guiding behavior change, and the need to adopt a co-operative approach to problem solving. We believe that it enhances clients' hope and self-efficacy to point out that they possess the skills to control their own behavior and that the treatment will help bring those skills to bear on their gambling.

Secure personal and gambling histories. In addition to an abbreviated version of a typical personal and social history, learn about the client's gambling experience. This history should include: age when first gambled, gambling experience growing up, changes in gambling behavior over time, any periods of abstinence, and preferences for types of gambling. In addition, ask clients to describe a typical gambling session. Listen for triggers, consequences, gambling-related irrational beliefs, and patterns of play. Find out about previous efforts to control their gambling, if such efforts have been made.

Be careful not to overlook possible comorbidity issues. In particular, it is important to ask about current and historical use of drugs and alcohol. As noted in Chapter 3, thorough assessment of depression is needed. A consideration of possible legal trouble, marital problems, and work performance is also valuable.

An initial consideration of positives and negatives. Next we encourage clients to begin a cognitive appraisal of the costs and benefits of change. Using reflective statements, you can have clients return to their reasons for seeking treatment. Information from the gambling history can also be helpful in encouraging the client to consider what is enjoyable and what is objectionable about gambling. In the same manner, clients also consider the potential positives and negatives associated with changing their gambling behavior. The objective with this preliminary Decisional Balance exercise is not to reach any decisions or commitments, but rather to begin to explore ambivalence around change. The hope is that clients will begin to develop a more complete picture of the consequences around change and failure to change. It is important not to let clients ignore either the positives or the negatives of gambling. It is very helpful for the person to consider that gambling has a beneficial side and that giving it up will have costs. Watch for clients taking short cuts by simply equating the costs of continuing to gamble with the benefits of change. While overlap is likely, there are also likely to be unique aspects to each set of positives and negatives.

Completion of assessment measures. Once the preliminary decisional balance discussion concludes, it is a good time to transition to completion of the assessment instruments. For the GSCG treatment, the G-TLFB, or Gambling Timeline Follow-Back, is the most important assessment measure. As previously described, you need to assist the client with the first month of the G-TLFB. Clients who bring an appointment book or bank statement often find that the calendar is not difficult to complete. Other clients are challenged by the task. Once the first month is completed the task usually becomes less daunting.

Other measures can be administered following the timeline. We typically administer the South Oaks Gambling Screen, Gamblers Belief Questionnaire, Gambling Self-Efficacy Questionnaire, Alcohol Use Disorders Identification Test, a marital satisfaction questionnaire, and a brief set of questions about income and expenses. We find it helpful and motivating to let the client know that they will receive feedback on each of these measures in the second session.

Homework. Once the assessment information is in hand, we meet again with the client to review the homework for the week. Descriptions of the homework assignments follow. Copies of all homework assignments appear in Chapter 8.

Mt. Recovery reading. This pamphlet, included in the toolbox (Appendix 5), provides a brief overview of overcoming a gambling problem and how to handle possible slips along the way.

Making a decision exercise. The decisional balance exercise is included in the toolbox (see Appendix 6). It offers the client a formal opportunity to evaluate the pros and cons of changing and not changing gambling behavior. It allows the client to see a full range of pros and cons and to avoid biasing or discounting positives and negatives that could affect the decision to change.

4.1.3 Phase 2: Motivational Feedback

During Phase 2 participants are provided with individualized feedback based on information obtained during the assessment phase. This feedback is designed to help clients recognize their high-risk behavior and to evaluate the extent to which gambling has negatively impacted their lives. A key element to this feedback phase is the use of information from the G-TLFB calendar to provide a detailed picture of recent gambling history. Clients are prompted to compare their recent gambling behavior to their "ideal" behavior as well as to levels of gambling in the general population. To further increase their motivation to change their gambling, we use the decisional balance homework described earlier.

Communicating the assessment results

Components of Phase 2

Review any recent gambling. Start the session, as you will every session, by reviewing any gambling episodes since the past meeting. The therapist should listen for any gambling-related events that might relate to the content of this treatment phase.

Feedback about client's gambling and its effects. The information collected from the Gambling Timeline Follow-Back and all other assessment measures is used to generate a feedback report. This report should be simple and use attention-grabbing graphs and tables to provide clients with detailed information related to their gambling. A sample report accompanies the case detailed in Chapter 5. Feedback should be provided for all measures the client completed. The feedback on some measures, particularly the Gambling Timeline Follow-Back, is useful in this phase as it can enhance motivation for change and establish a treatment goal. Other information in the feedback report is used in a later phase. For example, the GBQ information about irrational beliefs will be helpful when examining the role of these cognitions in initiating or maintaining a gambling session.

Clinical Pearl
Feedback Sessions

During feedback clients should be asked to do the following:

- Contrast their intent to risk money gambling with actual money wagered.
- Examine and describe monthly and daily gambling patterns.
- List other things that they could have done with money that they wagered.
- List other ways they could have spent time devoted to gambling.
- Discuss how the way they use their time is an accurate or inaccurate reflection of their priorities.
- Discuss how the way they spend their money gambling and in other areas (e.g., housing, food) is an accurate or inaccurate reflection of their priorities.
- Evaluate whether they can afford to keep up their current rate of gambling when gambling expenditures are extrapolated out into the future.
- Compare their SOGS score to a distribution of SOGS scores in the general population.
- Consider their scores on the measures of gambling-related irrational beliefs, self-efficacy to control their gambling, alcohol problems, and, if appropriate, relationship satisfaction with their spouse or significant other.

> **Clinical Pearl**
> **Maximizing the Motivational Impact of Feedback**
>
> To maximize the motivational impact of the feedback therapists should do the following:
>
> - Take your time to ensure that the client understands the feedback data.
> - Avoid interpreting clients' GTLFB data for them.
> - Ask open-ended questions.
> - Monitor client resistance during the feedback session and, when present, roll with it. Never actively confront resistance.
> - Listen for clients' statements that indicate a desire to change their gambling and use reflective statements to further reinforce motivation for change.

We slowly walk the client through the report and in a nonjudgmental manner focus the client on the information provided (e.g., gambling patterns, frequencies, expenditures). Remind clients that the report is derived from their responses to the questionnaires they previously completed. Emphasize that the goal of this feedback is not to make them feel guilty regarding their previous behavior, but instead, to provide them with information to let them know where they are and to help them make informed decisions regarding their gambling behavior. For example:

"The goal here is not for you to feel bad about what you have done in the past, but to get a better sense of where you are and to help you make better and more informed decisions about changing your gambling."

Consistent with the motivational perspective, the client should be primarily responsible for generating the interpretation of data presented in the feedback session. In order to encourage this, clients should be asked to contrast their past or current behavior with the desired behavior. In addition, they should be able to compare their behavior with normative data, and recognize the difference between their level of gambling and that of the general population.

Review decisional balance exercise. If a homework assignment was not completed prior to the session, complete it during the session. Incomplete decisional balance assignments are not unusual. Typically, clients will disclose that they had thought about the issues, but did not write their ideas on paper. You should accept such statements and then offer to assist the client with the exercise. While reviewing the assignment, have the client discuss the identified pros and cons of maintaining versus changing gambling behavior. Often it is valuable to individually list items that the client has placed in each category, and have them discuss the reasons for identifying these particular costs and benefits. You should also help the client generate additional items. Although therapists can and should ask "leading" questions, it is important that the client generate the items. Make sure that the client has listed items in each category. It is possible that a client may say "I do not see any benefits of continuing my gambling" or "I just can't think of any costs of stopping gambling since nothing but bad will happen if I continue." Help the client to understand the importance of identifying items in each outcome category by continuing to pose questions. Finally, as shown in Figure 3, we use a balance beam scale to help the client describe their decision about continuing or changing their gambling.

> **Draw your own scale**
>
> Now that you have thought about the costs and benefits of changing your gambling, take a few minutes to draw a scale that represents where you are right now. Please look over the examples on this page and the next and then draw your own scale.
>
> For example, if the costs and benefits of changing your gambling are about equal to the costs and benefits of not changing, then you would draw a scale like the one here:
>
>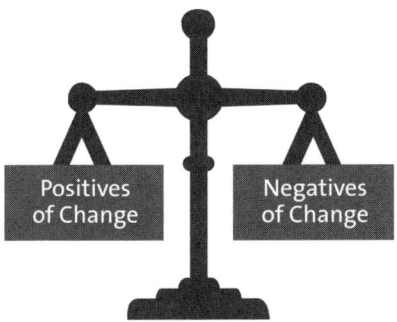
>
> **Figure 3**
> Balance beam scale used in the decisional balance exercise.

Goal statement form. Discuss the value of the client selecting his or her own treatment goal. We want the client to take responsibility for the change process and we assume that ownership of the goal increases motivation to change. Also note that the goal will be revisited each week and can change over time in response to experiences both within and between appointments.

As can be seen on the Goal Statement Form provided in the toolbox (Appendix 4), the client chooses between abstaining from gambling or gambling in some controlled manner. If a control goal is selected, the client needs to specify the gambling time and money limits. Encourage the client to explain the goal to you. The client should have solid reasons for choosing the goal. If the client does not provide adequate justification for the goal, query him or her as to why the goal was selected. It the goal is a controlled goal, it may be helpful to refer back to the information on the feedback report.

Review Mt. Recovery reading. The purpose of the Mt. Recovery reading is to help the client adopt a long-term perspective on changing gambling behavior. When discussing readings or homework with clients, remember that the interaction is conducted within a motivational framework. The goal is to help the client understand that changing one's gambling behavior is not often a simple or speedy task. Be sure to emphasize the importance of treating slips as learning experiences and provide a brief discussion of the abstinence violation effect. The abstinence violation effect is a feeling of loss of control that arises after a period of abstinence is broken. The perceived loss of control often results in the individual abandoning the belief that addictive behavior can be successfully changed.

Homework. Provide the client with the triggers and consequences homework (see Appendix 7), and ask them to complete it prior to Phase 3. Inform

Client selects treatment goal

> **Clinical Pearl**
> **Mt. Recovery Homework Review**
>
> Be sure to emphasize the importance of treating slips as learning experiences and provide a brief discussion of the abstinence violation effect. For example:
>
> - The purpose of this reading was to consider a long-term perspective on changing your gambling behavior.
> - While it would be great to change your gambling overnight, for most it is a slower process.
> - Ideally, you will never again gamble more than you intend, but if you should have a slip or exceed your goal, this does not constitute a failure!
> - We can use such situations as learning experiences rather than self-fulfilling prophecies of failure.

the client that the purpose of the exercise is to begin to understand the role of gambling in his or her life by assisting in the identification and understanding of high-risk gambling situations.

4.1.4 Phase 3: Triggers and Consequences

Conducting a functional analysis

During Phase 3, clients are guided through a functional analysis of their problematic gambling behavior. They are helped to identify specific triggers and consequences of their gambling behavior, as well as the role of these triggers and consequences in the initiation and maintenance of the behavior. It is during this phase that the role of gambling-related irrational beliefs in problematic gambling is introduced and discussed. Through this process, clients are better able to identify future situations that pose a risk for engaging in problematic gambling. This phase and the next are crucial skill building phases and client mastery is important.

Components of Phase 3

Review any recent gambling behavior. Review any gambling episodes since the past session. Refer back to the client's goal statement form and in a nonjudgmental manner address how any gambling might relate to the treatment goal. You might ask, *"How does your gambling over the past week fit with your goal?"* Invite the client to reconsider the goal. It is not uncommon for clients who choose a controlled goal to shift to an abstinence goal during treatment. As with the previous phase, note any element of the gambling that might relate to the content of this treatment phase.

Triggers and Consequences homework. Probe the client's understanding of the Triggers and Consequences homework. The client should understand that the reasons why people gamble can be explained by two sets of variables, triggers and consequences.

Triggers, or antecedents, are events that lead to gambling and can include situations, behaviors, thoughts, and emotions. If identified triggers are not specific, as is often the case, lead the client to identify triggers as specifically as possible. Use the Gambling Timeline Follow-Back to help the client remember specific gambling events and recall antecedents to the gambling.

When discussing triggers, spend time on the idea of gambling-related irrational beliefs. The Gamblers Beliefs Questionnaire can be very helpful in initiating this discussion. Traditional cognitive restructuring exercises can help the client understand how to eliminate some of the cognitive distortions that precipitate gambling episodes.

Work with the client to categorize individual triggers into categories that share common themes. These categories can be characterized as "typical problem gambling situations." If you must help the client to see common themes, here is an example of a useful prompt:

"When I look at the triggers you listed, two or three categories of triggers seem to stick out. These are situations in which you are angry or frustrated and days when you have some extra cash. Do you see the same things?"

Consequences are the results of gambling and can be either immediate or delayed. In the same manner used to identify triggers, have the client describe consequences and ensure that they are specific, representative of the gambling experiences, and important to the client. Sometimes clients will say, "There are no positive consequences of my gambling." Discuss possible examples with them such as feelings of winning, being able to "escape" from problems, or having fun. Contrast the difference between short-term and long-term consequences. As with many problematic behaviors, the immediate consequences of gambling are typically positive, while the more distant consequences are negative. Help the client to recognize this difference and the role that they play in the maintenance of gambling.

As with most aspects of this program, the goal is for the client to be responsible for generating the triggers and consequences. As the therapist, you can and should ask leading questions but should work hard to refrain from completing the functional analysis for the client.

Homework. Although titled "Dealing with Your Problem Gambling," we refer to the next assignment as the "Options Homework" (see Appendix 8). The goal of the homework is to generate options to gambling based on the functional analysis. We begin by offering the client a brief explanation for completing the assignment. Detailed instructions are printed on the homework sheet. Prior to giving the client the homework, you should have the client fill in the identified triggering categories in the blank space beside the "problem gambling situation" on each worksheet page.

"I want you to take the three general categories of triggering situations that we identified today and, in this exercise, identify alternatives and options to these high-risk situations that trigger your gambling."

4.1.5 Phase 4: Options and Action Plan

Phase 4 builds on skills learned and refined during Phase 3. During this phase, we highlight the importance of developing beneficial alternative ways to respond to environmental, behavioral, cognitive, and emotional events that serve as triggers for problematic gambling behavior. Throughout Phase 4, you should assist the client to identify, problem-solve, and prepare to implement specific beneficial alternatives to the triggers related to problematic gambling behavior.

Enhancing skills to address the gambling

Components of Phase 4

Review any recent gambling behavior. Review any gambling episodes since the past meeting. Use recent events to rehearse the identification of triggers and consequences. Refer back to the client's goal statement form and, in a non-judgmental manner, address how any gambling might relate to the treatment goal. Be open to the possibility that the client may want to change the goal. As in the last phase, note any element of gambling events that might relate to the content of this treatment phase.

Options homework. Probe the client's understanding of the options exercise. The client should understand that a problem-solving approach to triggering events will be helpful in developing options. Review and implementation of this homework gives us an opportunity to reinforce the importance of specificity when identifying triggers and consequences.

We try to be aware that developing options is not easy and most clients struggle with finding valuable and rewarding options. Be honest with them. Few activities will replace the excitement of gambling. For example, casino gamblers will not easily replicate the experience of being in a stimulating setting where people bring you complimentary drinks and provide free or low cost meals and hotel rooms. Viable options need to supplant the gambling experience, not replicate it and, hopefully, move the client closer to his or her goals. This issue is most apparent when considering the relative consequences of the identified options compared to the consequences of gambling. Have the client think through the rationale for options. Both client and therapist need to realize that identifying options is a creative exercise. Implementing options is trial and error. This means that some options will work while others will be disappointing. Clients need to understand the value of identifying, attempting, and evaluating options.

It is crucial to help the client generate specific action plans for implementing alternative behaviors. These plans should be as specific as possible, and, when appropriate, the plan should detail specific behaviors, in specific situations, with specific people.

"Now that you have generated alternative ways of responding to triggering situations, it is important to develop a plan for putting these options into action. If you plan what to do in advance you are much more likely to do it when confronted with these situations, or challenges to your beliefs."

Query clients regarding what triggering situations they anticipate experiencing prior to the next session. Ask them about problematic situations they anticipate encountering and specifically how they plan on dealing with these situations.

"What specific risky situations do you think you might experience before we meet again? Based on what we talked about today, how do you plan on handling these situations?"

Discuss ways of responding to and modifying cognitive processes that have led to problematic gambling behavior. Query clients regarding the actual validity of the cognitive distortions they are exhibiting. It is often beneficial to model ways in which to challenge the cognitive distortion and then ask the client to do the same. Many times, some level of brief education of the client on such things as randomness, probability, the idea of independence of events, and the business aspects of most gambling venues is helpful in challenging beliefs that are specific to gambling. Dysfunctional beliefs about related situations (e.g., job pressures, marital conflict) can be approached in a similar manner. If necessary, additional sessions in this phase can be used to monitor implementations of options and to address additional triggers.

Homework. Phase 5 covers relapse prevention. In preparation for this phase, ask the client to generate a list of three high-risk situations for relapse that he or she may encounter in the future (see Appendix 9). These may be similar or different than previously identified. The identified situations will be used in a Phase 5 discussion regarding relapse prevention.

> *"You have made a lot of great changes in your gambling behavior over the time that we have been working together. What potential situations do you see in the future that will make it most difficult for you to keep up these changes? For your homework this week I would like you to come up with three situations before our next session in which you think it will be difficult for you to refrain from gambling or gambling more than you want to."*

4.1.6 Phase 5: Relapse Prevention

This final phase builds on Phase 3 and Phase 4 skills but with a focus on relapse prevention. Clients are encouraged to develop plans for handling future high-risk situations. The abstinence violation effect is addressed, and ways of handling potential slips are discussed.

Learning from slips

Components of Phase 5

Review any recent gambling behavior. Ask about any gambling episodes since the past meeting and discuss them as they relate to the client's treatment goal. Remain open to the possibility that the client may want to change the goal.

High-risk situations. Ask about the three high-risk situations generated in the homework and possible plans for handling these situations. Engage the client in developing options and action plans for handling these situations. Prompt discussion of the benefits of any changes in gambling behavior. Discuss how the client handled triggering situations that he or she may have encountered since the previous session. Use these situations and how the client managed them to reinforce competencies and plans developed in the previous phases. Have the client consider any potential changes to the action plans that need to be made as a result of these recent experiences.

Managing high-risk situations

> *"Did you experience any of the challenging situations that you thought you might come across? Were there other situations or events that we did not prepare for? How successful were you at implementing the options that we had discussed or developing plans for new situations? Based upon what you experienced, do you need to make any modifications to the action plans? If so, what are they?"*

Your role in the development of these options and action plans should be minimal. By this point in the program the client should be able on his or her own to generate these problem situations.

Review concepts described in Mt. Recovery reading. Remind the client about the Mt. Recovery homework and review possible reactions to lapses and warn about the abstinence violation effect. Stress the importance of treating potential slips as learning experiences and highlight the importance of resuming the process of recovery as soon as possible after a slip.

Consider the changes. Often it is helpful to bring with you a copy of the initial feedback form from Phase 2 and have the client note differences between former and current behavior. The purpose of this exercise is to allow the client to generate self-efficacy statements and to increase the client's motivation for continued gains following treatment.

4.1.7 Follow-Up

Both client and therapist should identify improvements in gambling behavior and increases in client self-efficacy to control gambling across the five phases. However, past reductions in gambling behavior may not hold up over time and, as a result, the client will often report feeling anxious about maintaining the improvements. Many therapists share this concern. Scheduling a follow-up session provides both client and therapist a clear contact point at a specified date. The timeframe for this follow-up is up to the client and therapist. A meeting one, three, or six months later often provides reassurance to both parties.

We use the follow-up to assess the client's gambling and their well-being in other areas of their life. With a brief, yet personal reminder note about the follow-up session, we ask the client to bring in a completed Gambling Timeline Follow-Up covering the time since the last meeting. This information allows the client to review any recent gambling behavior and begin to establish the agenda for the follow-up session. We allow the client's recent gambling to dictate the content of the session.

> **Clinical Pearl**
> **Follow-Up Sessions**
>
> The following issues are possible discussion points during any follow-up sessions:
> - Comparison and discrepancy between behavior and goal.
> - Implementation of options and action plans.
> - What worked and what needs to be modified?
> - Abstinence violation effect.
> - How were past slips handled?
> - What are the plans for potential future slips?
> - What additional high-risk situations have you identified since the end of treatment proper?
> - List the benefits of decreased gambling behavior. Again, it is helpful to produce for the client the initial feedback form from Phase 2. Have the client compare their current behavior with the information on the feedback form.
> - Use successful behavioral experience as a self-efficacy builder.
> - What does your success over the past month tell you about your ability to control your gambling?
> - How will you maintain your progress?

This follow-up session provides an opportunity to reinforce the client for abstinence or successfully controlled gambling behavior. If the client has failed to meet goals, reflect with him or her on any previous positive changes and focus the client on increasing the learned motivation for change. Emphasize applying skills to the change process in general and high-risk situations in particular. Share an optimistic perspective with the client.

4.2 Mechanisms of Action

There are several change mechanisms we see as important to this treatment. First, this treatment is designed to capitalize on what naturally sets the stage for positive, long-term behavioral change. It is likely that a traumatic event might result in brief but unstable change. For example, big losses at the poker table and threats of divorce by a spouse may lead to short-term changes that do not hold up over time. Researchers have learned that successful recovery from addiction typically includes a cognitive appraisal of the individual's current behavior against his or her values and preferred self-perceptions. This process can motivate self-directed change. Early in GSCG treatment clients are encouraged to consider these discrepancies and the possibility of changing them.

Second, an important element in this appraisal process is providing the client with feedback about his or her gambling. The information gathered by the Timeline Follow-Back provides a detailed, yet comprehensive description of the client's recent behavior (Sobell & Sobell, 1993). It is likely that the feedback report to the client was the first time that this person had ever viewed the investment in gambling or considered how his or her gambling problems compared to other gamblers. It has been our experience that this feedback can be an eye opening event when managed by an accepting nonjudgmental therapist.

Third, this change process is dependent on the therapist viewing motivation as a dynamic state that can be influenced. Miller and Rollnick (2002) argued convincingly that a commitment to change establishes a sufficient foundation for gaining control over problematic behavior. Ambivalence about the target behavior and resistance to change are normal, constitute an important obstacle to recovery, and can be resolved through a flexible alliance between client and therapist. The therapist's success in increasing the client's readiness for change is essential for change. We see the use of the motivational interviewing style as a key element in this change process.

Finally, the application of functional analysis in behavior therapy has a long and empirically supported history. Within the motivational style described here, and using readings and homework assignments, we take clients through a behavioral and cognitive analysis of the maintaining conditions of their gambling behavior. We then use this process to develop options for managing the antecedents and consequences of gambling.

Antecedents in our model can be environmental, behavioral, or cognitive events. This leads, in later phases of this intervention, to client-managed interventions that can involve problem solving, coping skill enhancement, and cognitive restructuring strategies as appropriate to the targets of change identified in the functional analysis.

4.3 Efficacy and Diagnosis

Based on one of most evaluated treatments for addictions

Guided Self-Change (GSC) is one of the most empirically supported brief treatments for addictive behavior, with seven clinical trials supporting its efficacy (for comprehensive review see Sobell & Sobell, 1998, 2005). Since the first clinical trial with problem drinkers, this treatment has been contrasted successfully to medication, validated cross-culturally, used effectively with adolescents, expanded to include social support, and used in group and individual formats with alcohol and drug abusers. GSC has also been evaluated within a stepped care treatment delivery trial (Breslin et al., 1999).

GSC approach has been shown to effectively treat individuals with severe drinking problems. Initially, this approach was developed for low severity problem drinkers. Since this first study found that drinking severity was unrelated to treatment outcome, the approach was subsequently evaluated with individuals with serious alcohol problems. This research found support for Guided Self-Change with severe problem drinkers and with problem drinkers across different settings with positive results (for review see Sobell & Sobell, 1998, 2005). The finding that brief treatments are effective for more severely dependant drinkers has been replicated (Edwards & Taylor, 1994; Project Match, 1998; Sobell et al., 1998). Despite the expectations that serious problems require lengthier, more intense treatment, each of these studies found that response to treatment was unrelated to treatment length regardless of problem severity.

Our GSCG treatment is modeled after the Sobells' treatment, but has gone through a series of revisions in response to feedback from clients and therapists (Meyers, May, Steenbergh, & Whelan, 2000). While the objectives of the treatment have remained consistent with the model, treatment details have evolved. The assessment process has been streamlined to increase efficiency while still assessing all gambling domains of interest. The motivational feedback provided to clients has been modified to take advantage of the specific gambling information offered by the Gambling Timeline Follow-Back and to optimize motivational impact. The session content and homework exercises have been modified to increase treatment compliance. During Phase 3 we often consider gambling-related irrational believes as antecedents to gambling episodes and as a factor that might extend gambling episodes. The treatment content has evolved to include the issues and problems that pertain specifically to gambling.

The efficacy of our treatment has been piloted in a project with 36 consecutive clients who presented for treatment at our clinic (Meyers et al., 2000). Eleven (30%) of these participants dropped out of treatment and no posttreatment or follow-up gambling data were collected on these individuals. The assessment and treatment protocols were similar to the one described in this book. Clinical psychology doctoral students, who had completed our treatment training protocol, provided treatment under supervision. Table 7 presents posttreatment, pretreatment, and 9-month follow-up information on three problem gamblers and 22 pathological gamblers who completed treatment. All reported significant distress due to their gambling. Almost half were female and 28% were African-American. Although diagnostic interviews were not conducted with this sample, the average self-reported level of distress was typical for an individual present-

Table 7
Pretreatment, Posttreatment, and Follow-Up Information on The Gambling Clinic Clients

Measure	Pretreatment M (SD)	Posttreatment M (SD)	Follow-up M (SD)
South Oaks Gambling Screen	12.5 (4.4)	–	4.5 (2.9)
DSM-IV-TR symptoms[1]	6.6 (1.4)	–	1.2 (1.2)
% days gambling	18.3% (18.0)	3.9% (3.2)	3.2% (3.5)
Amount risked per gambling session	$897 (1058)	$241 (573.0)	$374 (621.7)
Average monthly gambling expenditure	$504 (574.4)	$81 (109.9)	$92 (230.0)

[1] A score of 5 or more indicates that the client met criteria for pathological gambling.

ing for outpatient psychological treatment. Three clients reported symptoms consistent with problem drinking and one reported a drug-use history.

At the follow-up, no participant met criteria for pathological gambling when considering the gambling symptoms for the previous six months. Comparing the pretreatment and follow-up G-TLFB data, clients reported an average 82.5% decrease in days gambling, an average 58.3% decrease in the amount of money risked per gambling session, and an average 81.7% reduction in monthly gambling expenditures. Levels of distress significantly decreased by the end of treatment, and these decreases were maintained out to the 6- to 9-month follow-up. Two out of three who reported heavy drinking at pretreatment assessment reported significantly decreased alcohol consumption at pretreatment and follow-up. Outcome was not related to demographic variables, including sex and ethnicity.

4.4 Variations and Combination Methods

As noted above, Mark and Linda Sobell and their colleagues have support for a number of variations of the Guided Self-Change approach. Most of these treatment variations have not yet been attempted with problem and pathological gamblers. Our experience adapting this approach for the treatment of gambling problems has lead to the exploration of two variations. For each of these variations we have examined the outcome (e.g., maintenance of change in gambling behavior) with multiple clients.

The first variation is using the treatment with couples. Marriages and committed relationships are very likely to be affected when one of the pair has a gambling problem. In addition, we have discovered that couples often gamble together. Although only one might be described as a problem or pathological gambler, the gambling is a valued activity that both enjoy. We have had several cases where we used GSCG as conjoint therapy. To date this has been very suc-

Working with couples

cessful and typically we find motivation for change is facilitated by the support of the spouse. In situations where only one member presents with significant problems, the conjoint therapy appears to promote couple's adoption of active, enjoyable options to gambling. It is very likely that the success of this variation is related to pretreatment marital satisfaction. We do not yet have enough experience with the conjoint treatment to understand the relationship between marital satisfaction and treatment success.

Address co-occurring alcohol and gambling problems

A second variation is using the treatment with individuals with comorbid gambling and alcohol problems. As described in Chapter 1, the rates of lifetime and current alcohol problems among those with gambling problems is quite high (e.g., Petry & Pietrzak, 2004). Because of the origins of this treatment, our Guided Self-Change approach to gambling problems is likely to have some effect on our clients' alcohol consumption as well as their gambling. For a number of clients we have learned of a coexisting alcohol problem during the running start assessment. We provide these clients with feedback on their alcohol consumption during the feedback phase. For some, we decided to focus the treatment only on gambling and do not directly address alcohol consumption (Lipinski, Whelan, & Meyers, in press). When we do this we see some reduction in the alcohol consumption from pretreatment to posttreatment. For others we encourage them to consider their alcohol consumption as well as their gambling as they proceed through the treatment program. We have found that this approach has also worked in reducing alcohol problems as well as gambling problems. For those who complete treatment we find reductions in gambling and in alcohol consumption that are maintained for at least six months.

We have good reason to believe there are benefits to combining GSCG with other treatments. In addition to alcohol problems, individuals with gambling problems often present with depression, marital and financial problems. While for some clients the depression abates, sometimes dramatically during treatment, others continue to struggle. This appears particularly true for individuals who have experienced a loss or trauma that predated their gambling problems. We do not address the depression directly within treatment. Instead, we refer these individuals to other professional options to concentrate on the depression or trauma. We have adopted a similar position for marital or relationship problems. We treat the gambling with GSCG and then encourage additional treatment or social support for the couple's problems. If the client is not being treated within a research protocol, we do not discourage adjunctive treatment with another professional as long as our client agrees to our open communication with other treating professionals. As for financial problems, we refer these clients to professionals who can advise them about addressing their debts and money management.

Another option for some patients is Gamblers Anonymous (GA). Meetings are available in larger cities, but not outside these urban areas. Some of our clients have previously attended GA and have decided not to continue to attend. Unless they are participating in a treatment protocol that requires isolation of our treatment, we do not discourage our clients from exploring GA, but we do not prescribe it. It is up to the client to decide. Currently we do not have evidence on the effect of GA on our clients.

4.5   Problems in Carrying Out Treatment

Most of our treatment challenges fall into one of two categories: client expectations and treatment integrity. By client expectations we mean client concerns, beliefs, or hopes that are inconsistent with our treatment approach. Education about the treatment that occurs in the first session typically helps the therapist and client better understand each other's expectations. However, there will always be people with unspoken preferences that do not fit with the model. For example, within the GSCG approach we are very unlikely to spend much time exploring possible historical factors that lead to gambling excess.

Other client expectation challenges are related to addictive behaviors, if not specifically gambling problems. One challenge that is quite unique to gambling is the struggle to accept that changing their gambling means not being able to win back money that was lost. Occasionally, this realization means disclosing to others that money has been lost, debt has accumulated, or loans cannot be repaid. Rather than challenge the irrational thoughts about ever recovering this money, we believe it is best to listen closely to these concerns and discuss such concerns within the decisional balance exercise. After addressing the issue through the decisional balance exercise, a referral to a financial advisor to learn how to manage debt can be valuable to clients who present such concerns.

More common is for clients to hold expectations that gambling is caused by a disease or lack of a spiritual relationship. Both of these views can be accommodated within the GSCG treatment as the motivational interviewing style reminds the therapist to join with the client's views about problems and goals for change. The challenge for the therapist is that these clients may hold other expectations and beliefs about addictive behavior and behavior change. In such situations, we try to carefully monitor how clients process the information that we provide to them and we remain aware of where our approach does not fit with their expectations. For example, such clients expect more of a confrontational approach to relapse rather than our approach of listening and learning from such experiences.

The other challenge we face in delivering this intervention is maintaining treatment integrity. Following the lead of the Sobells, we prescribe a set of treatment guidelines rather than scripting the agenda of each session and spelling out the client–therapist interchange. At the same time, we try to remain focused on gambling, the five phases, and maintaining a commitment to brief treatment. Within every treatment phase, however, there are treatment integrity issues that challenge the therapist. One set of issues revolves around clients not completing the components of a treatment phase and therapists staying focused on the objectives of that phase. For example, the most frequent problem in Phase 1 is keeping clients motivated to complete the assessment. For this reason it is important to keep the assessment battery to a reasonable length and to consider using two sessions when necessary. The most frequent assessment difficulty involves the Gambling Timeline Follow-Back. This measure is essential to the feedback process. Some clients struggle to remember specifics of their gambling episodes. For these clients, a second assessment session might be needed and the client should be encouraged to bring memory aids, such as bank statements and appointment books, to the next appointment. The therapist might also need to facilitate the measure's completion using

Challenges with specific client issues

Challenges in treatment integrity

the strategies outlined in the Timeline manual (Sobell & Sobell, 1996). Other clients express their ambivalence when asked to recall their gambling history. It is scary for clients to face how much money or time has been lost gambling. For these clients it is essential to return to the basic motivational interviewing skills and join, rather than confront, their ambivalence. Enhancing the clients' understanding of the assessment's purpose and reassuring them that the therapist is not going to judge them and that the information is confidential helps such clients.

Another treatment integrity issue is allowing sessions to drift. Most of our clients present with other problems in their life; many of these are linked to their gambling. These other problems tend to pull the focus away from gambling. For example, Yvonne, the client we discuss in Chapters 2 and 3, expressed distress related to job and family demands. She also indicated that gambling was a way of escaping from this distress. The difficulty is for the therapist to gain relevant information about the job and family without shifting the treatment toward these problems. To successfully manage these situations, it is important that we keep the components of the current phase in mind. We try to listen and learn from our clients while always bringing the focus back to their gambling.

Finally, ambivalence to enter treatment tends to be high among individuals presenting with addictive behavior. Some individuals schedule an appointment, but then fail to appear for treatment. Others attend only a single session and never return. We have realized some success in maintaining attendance by taking a motivational approach in our interactions with clients. We listen for what lead them to contact us on that day. We offer to send them information about gambling problems and our self-change program. We acknowledge that change is a difficult decision that might take some further consideration. Helpful ideas about such motivational strategies can be found in the Substance Abuse and Mental Health Service Administration publication listed in Chapter 6.

4.6 Multicultural Issues

The addictions literature is becoming increasingly informed about ethnic and cultural issues that influence addictive behavior and its treatment (e.g., McNeese, 2005). Some treatment researchers have discussed how to blend together empirically supported treatments and culturally sensitive therapies (Wagner, 2003). Other results suggest that ethnic minority status does not appear related to ratings of therapeutic bonding or treatment outcome, but satisfaction with treatment does appear related to ethnicity (Tonigan, 2003). Continued efforts are needed as the role of other cultural variables – such as help-seeking beliefs, acculturation, and perceived discrimination – is not well understood. Our knowledge of the relationship between these cultural issues and gambling treatment is nascent. As mentioned in Chapter 1, ethnic minorities appear to be at greater risk for gambling problems. The implications of this increased risk on treatment models are not clear.

We do have some support for effectiveness of GSCG treatment with members of diverse ethnic and cultural groups. Guided Self-Change treatment for alcohol has been translated into Spanish and evaluated in a study completed in Mexico. The Mexico project (Ayala, Echeverria, Sobell, & Sobell, 1998) supported the use of this treatment approach with this population, but also revealed that Mexican men were unwilling to participate in a group treatment condition. The treatment has also been successfully implemented with Hispanic adults and Hispanic and African-American adolescents (Sobell & Sobell, 2005). As for GSCG treatment, about 30% of problem gamblers presenting to our clinic are African-American and we have not detected a differences in response to treatment based on ethnic status of the client or the therapist (Meyers et al., 2000).

5

Case Vignette

The following is a summary of our treatment of Ryan. Please understand that this and all other names are fictional and we have changed elements in our description to protect Ryan's identity. However, this case represents an individual who presented himself for treatment at The Gambling Clinic (TGC) at the University of Memphis. The five phases of treatment were completed in five sessions over a seven week period. In addition, Ryan attended a follow-up session six months after the end of treatment.

5.1 Phase 1: Running Start Assessment

The assessment phase began with an unstructured discussion about what brought Ryan to our clinic. He admitted that he was there at his wife's insistence, but that he would keep an open mind about changing his gambling. We then provided a brief overview of the program as described in Chapter 4. A semistructured interview to collect a gambling history and basic demographic information followed. Like most who contact our clinic, Ryan was quite frank when talking about his gambling. This appointment was the first time he had ever sought help for gambling.

Ryan was a 44-year-old male who had been married for 17 years, lived with his wife and 15-year-old daughter, and worked as a site manager at a construction firm. He worked at the same company for 20 years and liked the work and his colleagues. For recreation and entertainment, he enjoyed camping. He and his family camped regularly with the same group of friends, frequently spring through fall. Ryan also enjoyed reading science fiction but had few other hobbies or interests. He reported no medical concerns and did not use medication on a regular basis. He was a daily cigarette smoker. Ryan did not drink alcohol, having stopped approximately 10 years ago after a minor automobile accident involving alcohol. Prior to the accident, Ryan "drank quite a bit" and "rarely went a day without a couple of beers." Ryan described himself as an early riser and reported no sleep problems.

Ryan began gambling at the casinos about 12 years ago but now more often plays electronic gaming machines in taverns. These machines encompassed a variety of games including slots, card games, and matching games. He reported playing the machines because "they're fun and entertaining," "they're exciting," and "they give me something to do." This was a recurrent theme for Ryan; he repeatedly referred to "entertainment" as a major reason for playing. Money, on the other hand, was not a critical motivator for his wagering.

Specifically, he reported making sure he "pays the bills first," risking only what he had available to lose, and didn't dip into other funds. Ryan visited the casino about once a month and played slots. During the past year, he had several big slots wins amounting to $18,000. Ryan reported current debt of $5,000 from his gambling. He reported an estimated total lifetime loss of $100,000.

A typical gambling session for Ryan began at the end of his workday, usually around 4:30 in the afternoon. On the drive home Ryan passed a local bar where friends and some family members typically congregated in the afternoons. He usually socialized briefly and then began playing one of the machines. While he played, he described feeling that he "wants to beat the machine" and that "it's more like a contest" than gambling. He usually spent between $50 and $200 and two to three hours in the bar. He reported playing as long as eight hours and losing as much as $1,300. Ryan described the bar as a place where he could always go to socialize with people he grew up with.

Ryan's wife, Doris, placed the original call to our clinic seeking information about services for her husband. During this initial contact, Doris informed the therapist that Ryan "would lie and not tell you anything about his gambling" and would "probably not be very helpful" but that she would encourage him to consider treatment. Eventually, Ryan called and made an appointment to come to the clinic. At this first appointment Ryan appeared motivated to change his gambling but the source of his motivation was unclear. His relationship with his wife appeared strained at times and he reported that gambling was a way to escape from her and be alone.

In completing our brief decisional balance exercise in this first session, Ryan reported the following positives and negatives about gambling:

Positives: entertainment, chance of winning some money, escape "no time to think of anything else while I'm playing," social outlet

Negatives: my wife doesn't like it, loss of money, time spent gambling

Ryan was then given the first two homework assignments, the Mt. Recovery reading that helps clients reconceptualize and manage slips and lapses in a more productive manner, and a more formal decisional balance exercise that asks clients to examine the positives and negatives of giving up gambling and the positive and negatives of not changing their gambling. After the interview, Ryan remained to complete the G-TLFB and a packet of gambling specific assessment instruments. One month of Ryan's G-TLFB appears in Table 8. The instruments were later scored by the therapist and personalized feedback prepared for the second session. The first session required two hours to complete all of the components of this phase.

Comment

Given the importance of the development of motivation for change in the Guided Self-Change model, the fact that Ryan's wife, Doris, was the one who initiated the therapeutic contact raised concerns for us. Reported strains in the marital relationship were also issues we wanted to integrate into our case conceptualization. Alternatively, we viewed Ryan's ability to risk only what he "can afford to lose" and "pay the bills first" as indicators that he was already exerting some control over his gambling. His ability to give up alcohol use after a triggering incident some 10 years ago was another demonstration of self-efficacy that we planned to build on.

Table 8
One Month of Ryan's 6-Month Timeline Follow-Back

	Sunday	Monday	Tuesday	Wednesday	Thursday	Friday	Saturday
Date		1	2	3	4	5	6
Type		Video	Video	Video	Video	Video	
How long		2.0 hours	1.0 hours	2.0 hours	2.0 hours	2.5 hours	X
Intend		$50	$75	$100	$50	$100	
Risked		$100	$100	$150	$100	$100	
Win/loss		-$100	$0	$25	-$50	$25	
Drinks							
Special day							
Date	7	8	9	10	11	12	13
Type	Video	Video	Video	Video	Video	Video	SLOTS
How long	5.0 hours	2.0 hours	1.5 hours	1.0 hours	2.0 hours	1.5 hours	6.0 hours
Intend	$100	$200	$75	$100	$50	$100	$400
Risked	$200	$100	$75	$200	$50	$200	$400
Win/loss	$400	$100	$0	-$200	-$50	-$100	-$200
Drinks							
Special day							

Table 8 (continued)

Date	14	15	16	17	18	19	20
Type	X	Video	Video	Video	Video	Video	X
How long		3.0 hours	1.5 hours	2.0 hours	1.5 hours	1 hour	
Intend		$200	$75	$50	$150	$50	
Risked		$200	$100	$50	$150	$75	
Win/loss		-$100	-$50	-$50	$100	-$25	
Drinks							
Special day							

Date	21	22	23	24	25	26	27
Type	X	Video	Video	X	Video	Video	X
How long		2.0 hours	2.0 hours		3.0 hours	2.0 hours	
Intend		$150	$150		$200	$200	
Risked		$100	$150		$250	$100	
Win/loss		-$100	-$50		$0	-$50	
Drinks							
Special day							

Date	28	29	30				
Type	X	Video	X				
How long		2.0 hours					
Intend		$125					
Risked		$125					
Win/loss		-$75					
Drinks							
Special day							

5.2 Phase 2: Motivation and Feedback

We began by inquiring about Ryan's week, one in which he "did not gamble" (except for the event noted below) and successfully resisted several urges to gamble. We then reviewed the two homework assignments Ryan had completed. Working within the motivational interviewing style, we confirmed that Ryan understood the content of the Mt. Recovery homework, that there is a possibility of slips, and that such events could serve as learning experiences for future success.

The decisional balance exercise was reviewed in session and Ryan provided a few examples of the pros and cons of both continuing to gamble and changing his gambling behavior. The therapist provided prompts and queries in order to clarify and reinforce Ryan's recognition of his reasons for and against changing his gambling. Like many clients, Ryan attempted to deny the benefits of gambling and the costs of changing. Using the motivational style, the therapist worked to ensure that Ryan recognized that there was a positive value to his gambling. This is intended to help the client recognize that there are attributes of gambling that are valued and that would likely be missed when removed. This information is also useful when conducting a functional analysis in Phase 3 and identifying high-risk situations in Phase 5. Table 9 contains examples of Ryan's identified costs and benefits of gambling and change.

Table 9
Costs and Benefits of Changing Versus Not Changing his Gambling

Benefits of changing	Benefits of not changing
• Reducing wife's complaints	• Escaping from wife's control
• Helping the marriage	• Socializing in the bar
• Quit losing money	• Enjoying the games
• More time for other activities	• Chance of a big win
Cost of changing	**Cost of not changing**
• Boredom	• Losing money
• No place to go after work	• Losing time
• No chance to win big money	• Fights with wife

In addition to the loss of time and money, Ryan was motivated to change by the fact that the games he played are no longer as entertaining as they once were. Ryan stated, "I just don't get as much out of it as I used to." When prompted, Ryan acknowledged that he was also motivated by his marital relationship. While Ryan saw his wife as "very controlling" and stated that she "wants to tell me what to do all the time," he wanted the relationship to improve and was willing to make some changes for it. He also pointed out that:

Ryan: If she were the only reason I'd still be gambling...
Therapist: Your wife is not the only reason for you to come here.

Ryan:	No, she wants me to come in but I'm here because I want to stop.
Therapist:	Why?
Ryan:	I'm ready to quit... It's sucked more lately. If I was spending money and getting anything back from it I probably wouldn't want to stop. But I don't get anything back from the money I spend.
Therapist:	Except pressure from your wife...
Ryan:	Yeah and that's not worth it...

Ryan reported that since the last session his wife organized a poker game with his family for small change. He enjoyed playing and stated that even though it was gambling, it didn't feel as though it was. He elaborated saying he would occasionally play poker for small stakes every once in awhile but never for much and that it was more of a social outlet.

Ryan:	Kind of ironic since she's the one that's trying to stop me from gambling.
Therapist:	She's the one that's encouraged you to stop gambling and she plans a night of gambling?
Ryan:	That's why it's not an issue of the gambling... it has to do with being in control.
Therapist:	By having you come here she is exerting control over you?
Ryan:	Uh huh. She wants to be able to control every situation she's in.
Therapist:	She wants to know where you are all the time?
Ryan:	No, it doesn't matter what it is, she just wants to get her two cents in.
Therapist:	She's trying to keep you from gambling just so she can be in control.
Ryan:	She doesn't care if I'm gambling or not. She wants me to be around more and not out spending her money or what she thinks is hers.
Therapist:	So your wife would like you to be around more.
Ryan:	Yeah... She'd like me to be around. I'd like to spend more time with my daughter but she's 15 and doesn't want to be with me at all. You know how that is.
Therapist:	Spending time with your daughter is important for you.
Ryan:	When her friends aren't around we have a good time together. When they are around she doesn't want to be with me but that's alright.
Therapist:	But your wife wants you around more even if it's just to keep tabs on you.
Ryan:	Well, maybe not just to keep tabs on me.

The session's primary focus was to review the assessment information gathered in Phase 1 in order to enhance Ryan's motivation to make changes. We used the feedback, most of which was taken from the G-TLFB, to place Ryan's gambling behavior in realistic contexts. This information also gave us opportunities to contrast his behavior with his stated goals and priorities. For example, in this and subsequent sessions we often asked Ryan if his gambling choices were consistent with his goals. In providing feedback, it was important to not pass judgment or comment on the gambling, but to ask Ryan for his reactions to and thoughts about the feedback. Table 10 contains the key pages of Ryan's individualized feedback report. As shown in this report, open-ended questions follow each piece of information provided to Ryan. As we walked Ryan through the information and these questions guided our discussion and his interpretation of the feedback. Our challenge is to monitor and manage resistance and ambivalence while using reflective statements to highlight and encourage any desire to change. We also provided Ryan information about his level of gambling problems, self-efficacy to control his gambling, level of irrational beliefs, and marital satisfaction. Ryan was not surprised by the financial results. Even with his lack of concern over financial consequences we took this opportunity to create motivation for change around finances.

Ryan: I've lost more on my 401k this year than gambling.

Therapist: The money doesn't seem to be as much of a concern?

Ryan: Yeah, I only spend money that I've got... I never spend money that needs to go to bills or anything.

Therapist: The money you spend on gambling is play money... money you can use for fun and so forth?

Ryan: Yeah the money is not as important. Of course at this point I could have spent it to get my RV fixed.

Therapist: Hmm...

Ryan: I've been planning to work on it myself since it'll be $150 to get it towed to the shop and probably $900 to get it fixed. I haven't had the time and with the money I've spent I could have easily had it towed to the shop and taken care of.

Therapist: The money you've spent gambling could have covered the repairs?

Ryan: Yeah, it's not that much work to get it done but I'd have to drain the gas out of the tank which I just had filled before the fuel pump broke so there's like 75 gallons of gas in it and obviously I can't do that.

Therapist: So I guess on some level the money lost from gambling does matter? You could be done with the RV and ready for summer camping.

Ryan: Yeah, I could have gotten it fixed instead of worrying about how I'd get it done myself. It's been sitting in my driveway for months.

Therapist: If you had the money available you might have gotten it fixed right away?

Ryan: Probably... I could have avoided the hassle if I still had the gambling money.

We then turned to the loss of time as a motivating factor for gambling change. Ryan was much more discouraged over the time he spent gambling than he was over his financial losses. "It becomes more real when I look at it like this." While he spent more time gambling at the bar than at the casinos he spent much more money during his few trips to the casinos. Finding better ways to utilize time would be a focus of future sessions. When asked about his results on the SOGS, Ryan reported: "I'm not surprised but I don't think I've really got that much of a problem. It's not really affecting me since I don't spend money that I don't have."

Table 10
Sample Pages From Ryan's Assessment Feedback Report

Facts about your gambling: A 6-month perspective

Intent: How much you intended to gamble

Over the course of 6 months *you gambled 141 times* and intended to wager $20,130. This is approximately 56% of your total reported income for this time period.

Risk: How much you wagered

Over the course of 6 months *you gambled 141 times* and actually wagered *$28,135*. This is approximately 78% of your total reported income for this time period.
Over the past six months you wagered *$8,005* more than you intended.
You wagered what you intended on 81 of 141 gambling episodes during the past six months.
What are your impressions of this graph?

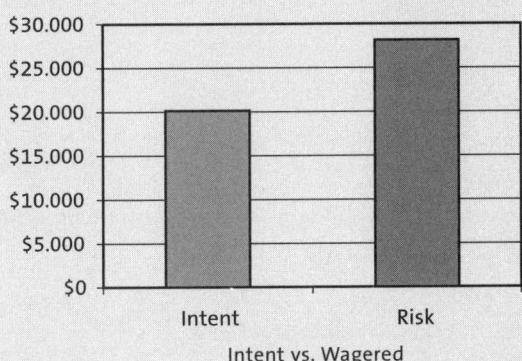
Intent vs. Wagered

Month by month overview of amount wagered

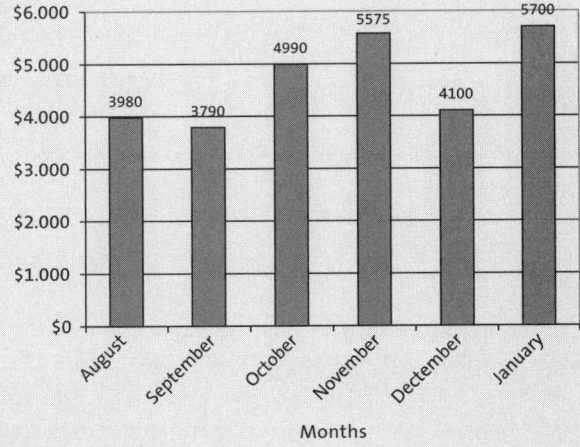
Months

What patterns do you see here?
What are some possible reasons why some months are greater than others?

Day by day overview of amount wagered

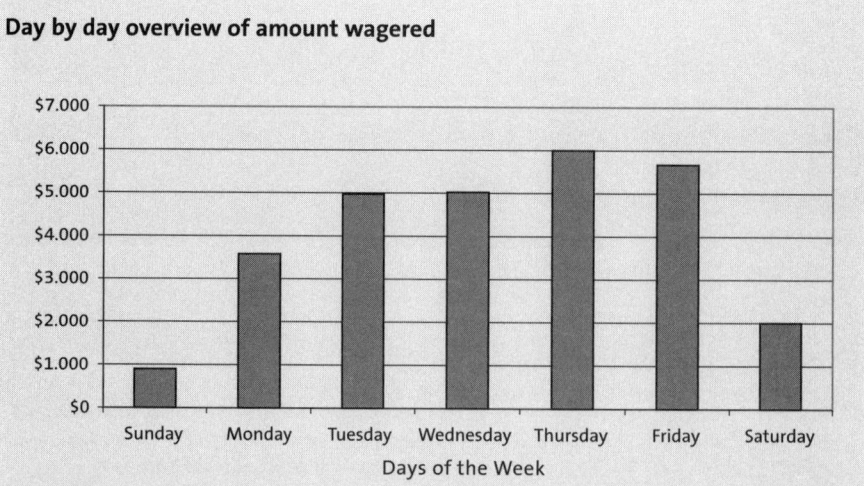

What patterns do you see here? Do you have any idea why some days are higher than others?
What are some other things that you could have done with that money you wagered?

Time: How much time you spend gambling

Over the past 6 months you have gambled about *292 hours or 12 days*.
What are some other things that you could have done with that time? Does the amount of time you spent gambling as compared to doing other things reflect your priorities? What's important to you?

Win/Loss: How much you won or lost gambling

Your gambling losses for the past 6 months totaled approximately *$5,945 or 29% of your income*.

If you continued with this current pattern of gambling, your losses would be:

Years	Projected Losses
1	$11,890
5	$59,450
10	$118,900
25	$297,250

If you had a job paying just $8 an hour during the hours you gambled, you would have earned *$2,336*. Instead, you lost about *$20* per hour gambling.

Compared to other major categories of financial expenditures in your life, housing, food, etc., gambling made up 31% of how much you spent over the past 6 months.

You told me about priorities. Does the way you spend money reflect your priorities in life? If someone were to view how you spent your money, would they get an accurate picture of those priorities?

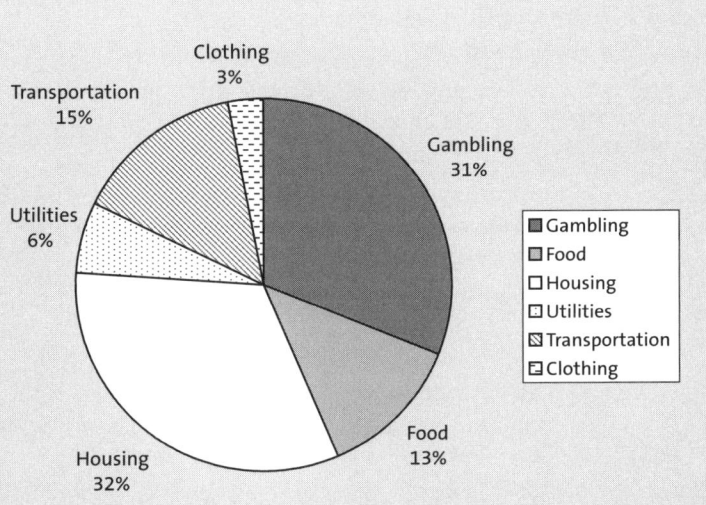

Where does your gambling fit in with others?

You scored 9 out of a possible 20 points on the South Oaks Gambling Screen (SOGS).

A score of 5 or greater is indicative of a potential pathological gambler. A pathological gambler is someone who experiences serious problems from gambling.

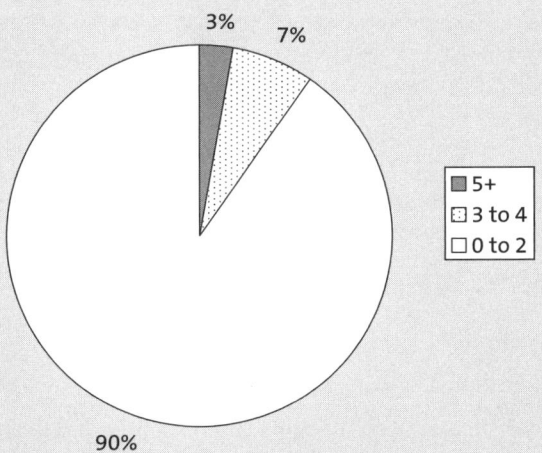

SOGS Score for Adult Male Population

As you can see only about 3% of the adult population scores 5 or above. What do you think about this?

Where does your drinking fit in with others?

You scored 0 out of a possible 40 points on the Alcohol Use Disorders Identification Test (AUDIT). Your AUDIT score shows whether your drinking should be considered a problem. A score of 8 or greater is indicative of a potential problem drinker. A problem drinker is someone who can experience serious problems from drinking.

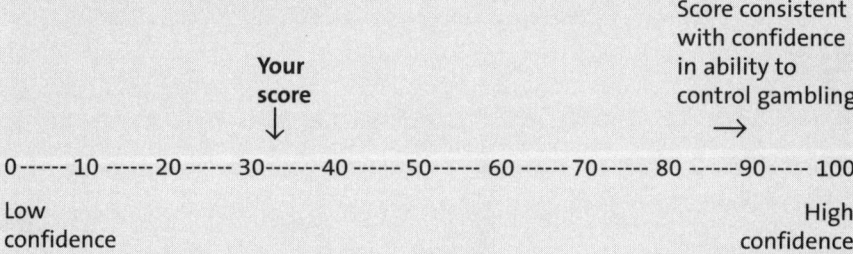

Your severity level : **0**

Level of risk for drinking problems
Low: 0–7
Medium: 8–15
High: 16–25
Very high: 26–40

What do you think about this? Is this consistent with your view of your drinking?

How confident are you about controlling your gambling?

You scored 31.25 out of a possible 100 points on the Gamblers' Self-Efficacy Questionnaire (GSEQ). A score of 100 means you are totally confident in your ability to control your gambling. A score of 0 means you have very little confidence in your ability to control your gambling.

Confidence to control gambling

```
                  Your                     Score consistent
                  score                    with confidence
                    ↓                      in ability to
                                           control gambling
                                                →
0------ 10 ------20 ------ 30--------40 ------ 50------ 60 ------ 70------ 80 ------90 ----- 100
Low                                                                              High
confidence                                                                       confidence
```

Most people who have not experienced problems due to their gambling tend to score above 85 on this measure. Your score is over 50 points lower than scores typically reported by problem-free gamblers.

How confident are you in your ability to control your gambling compared to others?

How your thoughts impact your gambling

Most people have superstitious thoughts when it comes to gambling, sometimes mistakenly believing they have control over events that they have no control over. Sometimes we all think that we can either detect when we are lucky or do things that make us lucky. Unfortunately, people who have many of these thoughts tend to gamble in ways that cause problems.

The Gamblers' Belief Questionnaire measures a person's level of such beliefs.

You scored *95* on the Gamblers' Beliefs Questionnaire (GBQ). People who gamble without problems almost always score less than 70 on this measure. People who have high levels of superstitious thinking may be prone to gambling problems.

5. Case Vignette

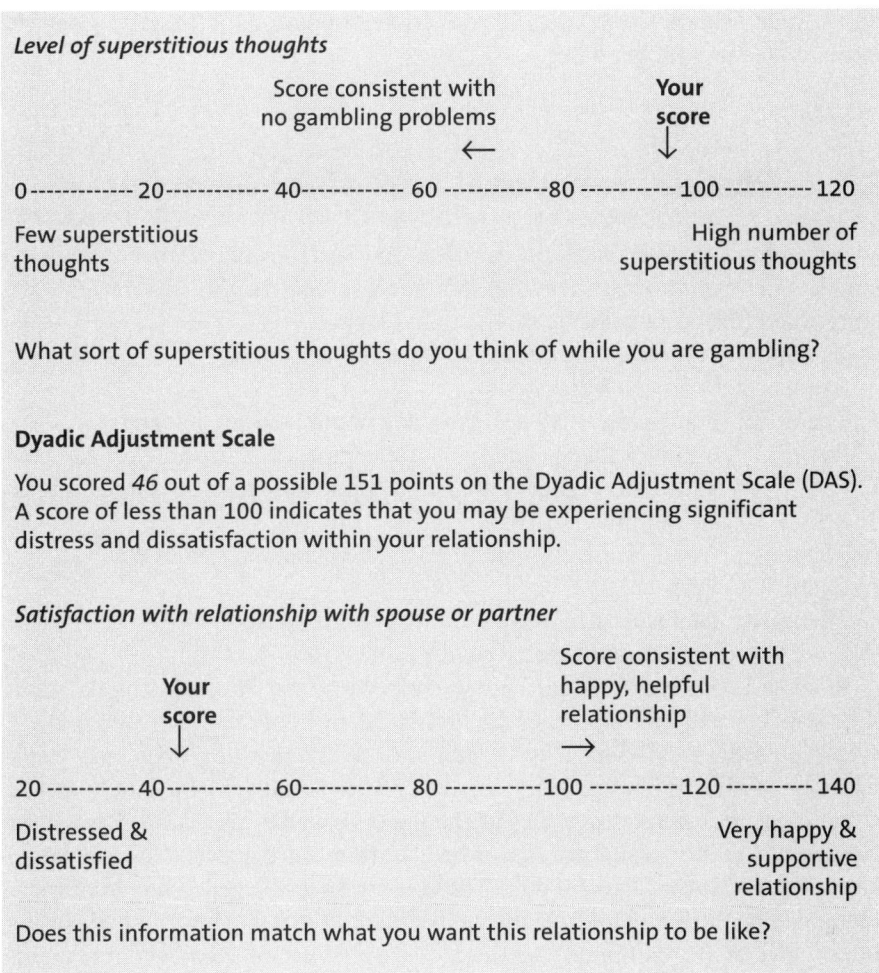

After receiving the feedback, Ryan completed the Goal Statement form. His reported goal was to reduce the time he spends gambling as, once again, he did not perceive the loss of money as a critical factor. In particular Ryan wanted to gamble for one to two hours and limit his spending to $100. He also hoped to reduce the number of days he plays each month to 15 from the current 25. Curiously, his gambling goal did not correspond with his last few weeks of abstinence from gambling. Ryan stated that this was because he had no intention of gambling and was very confident that he would stop. This was reflected in his rating of 100% confidence in reaching his goal. We gave Ryan the third homework assignment, Triggers and Consequences, to help him begin to conduct a functional analysis of his gambling behavior.

Comment

In this session we employed information gathered in the first session and from the assessment to focus Ryan on reasons to reconsider his gambling choices. This resulted in a less enthusiastic appraisal of gambling as entertainment, reaffirmation of time gambling as a serious problem, and recognition that gambling losses negatively impact Ryan and his family. Perhaps most importantly, Ryan acknowledged that he was driven, in part, by a desire to improve the relationship with his wife.

5.3   Phase 3: Functional Analysis of Gambling

Ryan reported that he had not gambled and had not experienced urges to gamble. His initial attribution for this success was largely external so we approached this issue with the motivational style.

Therapist: You haven't gambled in several weeks now.
Ryan: I've been busy at work.
Therapist: You haven't had any time you could stop by the bar?
Ryan: Actually I went into the bar this past week to show off my new truck. But I haven't wanted to gamble. I'm just not interested in it right now.
Therapist: Wow! You were able to go in there and not gamble?
Ryan: Yeah.
Therapist: That's great.
Ryan: Yeah, I don't really need it.

Ryan had completed the third homework. We began by discussing the gambling triggers and consequences he had listed in his homework assignment. Ryan reported his daily drive by the bar, not having anything to do, and wanting to escape his wife as primary triggers. He elaborated, "I'm usually awake at 5 o'clock in the morning. I read the paper, I watch television, I walk the dog and my family is still not out of bed for four more hours. I'm completely bored! What else do I have to do?" The consequences he generated were wasting money on the bar machines or casino slot machines that he could be putting into savings or into camping, spending too much time at the bar, and having his wife get angry and frustrated with him. The ensuing discussion was directed at fleshing out our understanding of the events that cued Ryan's gambling and developing a comprehensive picture of the consequences of those gambling episodes.

Ryan returned to the conflicts he had with his wife. He stated that she "provides no support" for him. It was apparent that he wanted to spend more time with Doris but now saw insurmountable barriers to this interaction. Even though Ryan had referred to the social aspects of gambling, playing the video machines had basically been a solo activity for him. Periodically he and his wife would go to the casinos together but this was rare.

Therapist: When you go to the casinos with friends what happens?
Ryan: I go down and spend time gambling and leave. It's not a problem.
Therapist: It's when you're alone that it becomes an issue?
Ryan: When I'm alone I don't have to worry about coming back with anyone, how much time I spend down there or how much money I spend. When I'm involved with others I'm not there as long. Even if I'm there with my wife, we can have fun.
Therapist: When you go with a group things are okay.
Ryan: Yeah. I need to watch out for that.

When we began discussing the issue of boredom, Ryan reported that his wife started having migraine headaches four years ago and her condition had forced her to stop working. As a result she has been on disability for the past eight months. She often goes through spells where she is disoriented and confused. This has left her irritable and, in turn, frustrates Ryan. He sometimes thinks she is lazy and will not work for herself and "uses it as a crutch." Ryan also stated that his wife is taking medicine that "takes away her appetite." This has led them to stop going out to breakfast and dinner, two activities that they previously enjoyed. Ryan said he would like to do more together but often fights with his wife. He reported wanting to plan an activity they could do together but that she is usually unwilling to go along or feels bad and cannot go.

Therapist: Wow… that sounds really frustrating. I guess it makes sense why you'd want to find a way to escape.

Ryan: Yeah, more often than not she's just sitting at home watching TV or sleeping.

Therapist: When you want to go out to do something…

Ryan: Even if I was there, she wouldn't want to go out or do anything.

Therapist: What would you like to do with her?

Ryan: We used to go out to breakfast on Saturday mornings. The three of us would all go out to eat for breakfast but since she often sleeps until 10:00 or 11:00 I don't have anything to do. Maybe I'll ask them to do that. If I tell them ahead of time they'd probably be willing to go.

Therapist: Sounds like a good way to do something together.

An examination of Ryan's gambling triggers and consequences helped us develop an initial hypothesis of a cycle of behavior that sustained Ryan's gambling. Boredom at home and the desire to limit contact with Doris when she was lethargic and negative produced an urge for escape and stimulation that typically resulted in a stop at the bar after work. As Ryan spent more time and money gambling, Doris's anger increased, creating a more negative atmosphere at home. The resulting tension between Ryan and his wife further limited any shared activity.

The remainder of the session was devoted to exploring these events and discussing how Ryan might manage them. Ryan was given the fourth homework, Options, which required him to formalize his plans for dealing with triggers.

Comment

The third session gave us a working model of Ryan's gambling. Our problem solving activities in the next two phases could now focus on generating alternatives to Ryan's gambling that might reduce his boredom, improve relationships at home, and moderate his need to "escape" from his wife. We also made an attempt to work with Ryan to allow him to take credit for the work he was doing in the therapy and gain a sense of efficacy for the significant changes he had made in his gambling.

5.4 Phase 4: Implementation of Alternative Behaviors

Ryan returned with his options homework completed. Again, he had not gambled and reported experiencing few urges to gamble. On the homework assignment, Ryan generated the following alternative responses to his triggers: cleaning his cars, camping in his RV, going somewhere in the mornings to read the paper such as a local coffee shop (something he enjoyed doing in the past), and spending more time with his family. This assignment proved to be particularly difficult for Ryan because he didn't have a lot of interests outside of camping and his social network revolved around the bar where he frequently gambled. Additionally, Ryan's marital troubles made working with his wife problematic. Because of this, we elaborated on the options he generated, examined their likely consequences and attempted to come up with additional strategies for dealing with free time and solutions for preventing and managing conflict at home. Ryan reported enjoying spending time with his wife but noted that their schedules often did not match or she was unwilling or unable to spend time with him. As such he found himself with a lot of time on his own. He also reported that he would like to spend more time with his daughter but understood that at 15 she is devoting her time to her peers. While frustrated with his wife, Ryan appeared interested in resuming some of the activities they had enjoyed in the past.

Therapist: So you've got a lot of empty time, Doris is usually in no mood to want to be with you and Samantha's pretty focused on her friends. But we've talked about a bunch of options. What do you think?

Ryan: I don't know if anything's going to change Doris.

Therapist: Then we're sort of stuck here.

Ryan: I know I've got to do something.

Therapist: What would you like to do? What activities might you and Doris do together?

Ryan: Well, you and I have talked about breakfast on Saturday mornings and I think that would work if I planned ahead and we went late enough.

Therapist: Right. What else? What about solutions that will work with Doris's migraines?

Ryan: Maybe in the evening I could rent a movie we'd both like to see. That way, even if she couldn't make it through the whole thing we could finish it the next day. Pick up some of her favorite foods. Stuff like that. She might like that and it would be a lot easier to be around her if she was in a good mood.

By session's end we had several options for each trigger identified in the previous session. We briefly discussed any triggering situations that might come up in the next week and how Ryan might apply some of the plans we made in the session. Then Ryan was given the last homework assignment in preparation for a discussion of relapse prevention in the final session. In this homework Ryan was asked to list three situations that could occur in the future that might place him at risk for possible relapse.

Comment

The options generated in this session were intended to give Ryan alternatives to gambling. In many cases, the alternatives were also intended to offer more positive interactions between Ryan and his wife, Ryan and his daughter, or among all three family members that might serve to prevent situations that could serve as prompts for gambling. The options also took into consideration the limitations imposed on Doris by her medical condition.

5.5 Phase 5: Relapse Prevention

The session began with an inquiry about any triggering situations that may have occurred during the week. We also asked about any new triggers or changes in Ryan's plans that might have taken place. Ryan did not gamble during the week but he did have an urge or two related to already identified triggers – boredom and frustration. He was able to manage these quite easily with family time and reading.

Ryan returned with the fifth homework completed. He reported three potential high-risk situations: having free time, going to Las Vegas for a conference, and feeling frustrated with his wife. He went on an annual week-long trip to Las Vegas and in the past had spent close to $4,000 gambling. To address this temptation, Ryan planned to stay with a group because he is better able to control his gambling when he is with others. Ryan felt that he would be able to maintain his goals because: "I've got my mind set on it and once I do that, I can quit whenever I want. It's just like when I quit drinking and never looked back."

We reviewed his initial Mt. Recovery homework and discussed the abstinence violation effect. We also reviewed in session his responses to the Gambling Self-Efficacy Questionnaire to further examine situations where he felt high versus low confidence about his ability to control his gambling. Even though Ryan had maintained abstinence since just before the first session, we discussed how he would interpret a potential slip and use the knowledge and skills he developed during our sessions to manage the situation.

We revisited Ryan's view of the benefits of changing his gambling behavior and we compared his responses to those he generated in the decisional balance exercise – reducing conflict with Doris, and having more time and money. To those Ryan now added a sense of confidence about his effort and a comfort that he was doing something he was proud of and that contributed to his family's well-being.

Ryan then completed another set of assessment materials and an appointment was made for the six-month follow-up session. He was reminded that he could contact the clinic if needed during the break and that we would call to remind him of the appointment.

Comment

In this session Ryan demonstrated an ability to independently generate plans for dealing with high risk situations for gambling, to understand the abstinence violation effect, and perhaps most importantly, to express a sense of self-efficacy about the changes he had made in his gambling behavior. Ryan continued to see his wife's moods and health condition as potential triggers for gambling. He recognized that these situations would produce a good deal of frustration and he would have to be prepared to manage them effectively. He seemed confident that he could do this.

5.6 Six Month Follow-up

Ryan reported that he had gambled once over the past six months. He went alone to a casino about three months ago on a Saturday afternoon. "I wanted to go and just see what it was like." Ryan reported having had previous urges to gamble but when such an urge came on he was quickly able to decide whether or not to act on it. "It's been easy to resist the urges... I just make a decision not to go." Ryan could not identify any specific triggering situations for this particular gambling event. He felt an urge and "just wanted to go." After further discussion he said, "I guess I was just bored and wanted to see what it would be like."

Ryan reported driving to the casino with $100 and planning to play up to $500 by using his two ATM cards to get another $400. After 40 minutes of playing $5 slots he won $1,500 and decided to leave the casino. Ryan described the gambling, even before the win, in this way.

Therapist: What was it like for you while you were gambling?
Ryan: It wasn't fun. I felt guilty, like I wasn't supposed to be here. It's hard to say this but I think I would've left even without the big win and maybe with at least some of my money left.
Therapist: So it really had an effect on you?
Ryan: Yeah, I felt bad the whole time and even the win only kicked up my spirits for a minute. I mean, it probably would have been better if I had lost because it would have at least justified the feelings. I was surprised how it wasn't any fun. The whole way home, I felt really guilty and angry.

Ryan reported having difficulty implementing some of his options because his wife had withdrawn even more over the past few months. She had recently started playing online poker (not for money) for three to four hours a night and sleeping until 11 or 12 in the morning. He stated that his options have had to change. He continued to spend a lot of time at work and going camping frequently, but has had to find things to do with his time in the morning when his family was not awake. "But I'd rather sit at home and be bored to tears than go back to the bar. I guess I didn't realize how much time I was spending there and how it was affecting me. Now I just feel a lot better about my life. Now I think I can see that I was probably a problem gambler. Maybe not like a lot of people because it didn't hurt my life and family that much except for the time I was spending." Ryan believed firmly in his responsibility to control his actions and that he was the one who had to make the tough decisions about his life. He believed that he could help his wife confront her gambling.

Ryan described his one gambling trip as a positive learning experience. He essentially described the event in relapse prevention terms. "I'm not going to let it make me feel like I'm back to square one" and "I'm not back to the beginning." Ryan remained highly motivated to reduce his gambling and noted many occasions during the past six months when he successfully resisted urges to gamble and used his plans to choose alternatives to gambling. He is concerned about his wife but he is committed to the marriage. Ryan was asked to complete the assessment battery and make an appointment for the one year follow-up. Ryan was again reminded that he could contact the clinic if needed and that we would contact him prior to the next follow-up.

Comment

Ryan appeared to have established a consistent and long-term control over his gambling. Importantly, he was very aware of this and appeared to take appropriate credit for this change. He knew that his wife's physical and psychological health, and her recent gambling, would continue to present challenges, but he seemed to have accepted this reality and actively planned to manage its effects on his choices around gambling. His efficacy for future control of his gambling was high.

6

Further Reading

This section includes key references to literature where the practitioner can find further details or background information.

Ladouceur, R., Sylvain, C., Boutin, C., & Doucet, C. (2002). *Understanding and treating pathological gambling*. West Sussex, England: Wiley & Sons.
  The authors' empirically supported cognitive treatment for problem and pathological gambling is presented. It also includes a review of the treatment literature, assessment methods, and responses to treatment difficulties.

Miller, W. R., & Rollnick, S. (2002). *Motivational interviewing: Preparing people to change addictive behavior* (2nd ed.). New York: Guilford Press.
  This volume contains theory and methods of motivational interviewing. It includes detailed descriptions of many practical techniques and procedures.

Petry, N. M. (2005). *Pathological gambling: Etiology, comorbidity, and treatment*. Washington, DC: American Psychological Association.
  Petry presents a comprehensive review of etiological factors and comorbid diagnoses. In addition, the author includes a detailed overview of treatment models with an emphasis on her cognitive-behavioral treatment for pathological gambling.

Sobell, M. B., & Sobell, L. C. (1993). *Problem drinkers: Guided self-change treatment*. New York: Guilford.

Sobell, M. B., & Sobell, L. C. (1998). Guiding self-change. In W. R. Miller & N. Heather (Eds.), *Treating addictive behaviours* (2nd ed., pp. 189–202). New York: Plenum.
  These two references provide the reader with greater detail about the Guided Self-Change approach to treating addictive behavior. Included are discussions of empirical support, treatment guidelines, and practical suggestions for using this treatment approach.

Substance Abuse and Mental Health Service Administration. (2000). *Enhancing motivation for change in substance abuse treatment*. Treatment improvement protocol (TIP) Series number 35. DHHD Pub No. (SMA) 00-34-60. Washington, DC: U.S. Government Printing Office.
  This volume is a helpful manual that details motivational strategies and ideas. Can be obtained free of charge from the National Clearinghouse for Alcohol and Drug Dependence by calling 1-800-729-6686 or go to http://www.ncbi.nlm.nih.gov/books/bv.fcgi?rid=hstat5.chapter.61302

References

Adamson, S. J., & Sellman, J. D. (2001). Drinking goal selection and treatment outcome in out-patients with mild-moderate alcohol dependence. *Drugs and Alcohol Review, 20*, 351–359.

Aczel, A. D. (2004) *Chance: A guide to gambling, love, the stock market, and just about everything else*. New York: Thunder's Mouth Press.

American Psychiatric Association. (1987). *Diagnostic and statistical manual of mental disorders* (3th ed.). Washington, DC: Author.

American Psychiatric Association. (2000). *Diagnostic and statistical manual of mental disorders* (4th ed., text revision). Washington, DC: Author.

Ayala, H. E., Echeveria, L., Sobell, M. B., & Sobell, L. C. (1998). An early and brief intervention alternative for problem drinkers in Mexico. *Acta Comportamentalia, 6*, 71–93.

Baker, T. B., Piper, M. E., McCarthy, D. E., Majeske, M. R., & Fiore, M. C. (2004). Addiction motivation reformulated: An affective processing model of negative reinforcement. *Psychological Review, 111*, 33–51.

Bandura, A. (1997). *Self-efficacy: The exercise of self-control*. New York: W. H. Freeman.

Barnes, G. M., Welte, J. W., Hoffman, J. H., & Dintcheff, B. A. (2005). Shared predictors of youthful gambling, substance abuse, and delinquency. *Psychology of Addictive Behaviors, 19*(2), 165–174.

Bechara, A. (2003). Risky business: Emotion, decision-making, and addiction. *Journal of Gambling Studies, 19*, 23–51.

Benshain, K., Taillefer, A., & Ladouceur, R. (2004). Awareness of independence of events and erroneous perceptions while gambling. *Addictive Behaviors, 29*, 399–404.

Black, D. W., & Moyer, T. (1998). Clinical features and psychiatric comorbidity of subjects with pathological gambling behavior. *Psychiatric Services, 49*, 1434–1439.

Bland, R. C., Newman, S. C., Orn, H., & Stebelsky, G. (1993). Epidemiology of pathological gambling in Edmonton. *Canadian Journal of Psychiatry, 38*, 108–112.

Blaszcznski, A. P., Huynh, S., Dumlao, V. J., & Farrell, E. (1998). Problem gambling within a Chinese speaking community. *Journal of Gambling Studies, 14*, 359–380.

Blaszczynski, A. P., Ladouceur, R., & Shaffer, H. J. (2004). A science-based framework for responsible gambling: The Reno model. *Journal of Gambling Studies, 20*, 301–317.

Blaszczynski, A. P., McConaghy, N., & Frankova, A. (1991). A comparison of relapsed and nonrelapsed abstinent pathological gamblers following behavioural treatment. *British Journal of Addiction, 86*, 1485–1489.

Blaszczynski, A. P., & Nower, L. (2002). A pathways model of problem and pathological gambling. *Addiction, 97*, 487–499.

Blum, K., Cull, J. G., Braverman, E. R., & Comings, D. E. (1996). Reward deficiency syndrome. *American Scientist, 84*, 132–145.

Breen, R. B., Krudelbach, N. G., & Walker, H. I. (2001). Cognitive changes in pathological gamblers following a 28-day inpatient program. *Psychology of Addictive Behavior, 15*, 246–248.

Breslin, F. C., Li, S., Sdao-Jarvie, K., Tupker, E., & Ittig-Deland, V. (2002). Brief treatment for young substance abusers: A pilot study in an addiction treatment setting. *Psychology of Addictive Behavior, 16*, 10–16.

Breslin, F. C., Sobell, M. B., Sobell, L. C., Cunningham, J. A., Sdao-Jarvie, K., & Borsoi, D. (1999). Problem drinkers: Evaluation of a stepped care approach. *Journal of Substance Abuse, 10*, 217–232.

Caron, A., & Ladouceur, R. (2003). Erroneous verbalizations and risk taking at video lotteries. *British Journal of Psychology, 94*, 189–194.

Cicchetti, D. (2006). Development and psychopathology. In D. Cicchetti & D. J. Cohen (Eds.), *Developmental Psychopathology: Theory and Method* (2nd ed., Vol. 1, pp. 1–23). New York: Wiley.

Comings, D. E., Gade-Andavolu, R., Gonzalez, N., Wu, S., Muhleman, D., Chen, C., et al. (2001). The additive effect of neurotransmitter genes in pathological gambling. *Clinical Genetics, 60*, 107–116.

Coventry, K. R., & Norman, A. C. (1998). Arousal, erroneous verbalizations, and the illusion of control during a computer-generated gambling task. *British Journal of Psychology, 89*, 629–645.

Cunningham-Williams, R. M., Cottler, L. B., Compton, W. M., & Spitznagel, E. L. (1998). Taking chances: Problem gamblers and mental health disorders: Results from the St. Louis Epidemiological Catchment Area (ECA) Study. *American Journal of Public Health, 88*, 1093–1096.

Curry, S. J., & Kim, E. L. (1999). Public health perspective on addictive behavior change interventions: Conceptual frameworks and guiding principles. In J. A. Tucker, D. M. Donovan, & G. A. Marlatt (eds.), *Changing addictive behavior: Bridging clinical and public health strategies* (pp. 221–250). New York: Guilford.

Davidson, G. C. (2000). Stepped care: Doing more with less. *Journal of Consulting and Clinical Psychology, 68*, 580–585.

Derevensky, J. L., Gupta, R., & Winters, K. (2003). Prevalence rates of youth gambling problems: Are the current rates inflated? *Journal of Gambling Studies, 19*, 405–425.

Dickerson, M. (2003). The evolving contribution of gambling research to addiction theory. *Addiction, 98*, 703.

Dickerson, M. G., Hinchy, J., & England, S. L. (1990). Minimal treatments and problem gamblers: A preliminary investigation. *Journal of Gambling Studies, 6*, 87–102.

Edwards, G., & Taylor, C. (1994). A test of the matching hypothesis: Alcohol dependence, intensity of treatment, and 12-month outcome. *Addiction, 89*, 553.

Eisen, S., Lin, N., Lyons, M. J., Scherrer, J. F., Griffith, K., True, W. R., Goldberg, J., & Tsuang, M. T. (1998). Familial influences on gambling behavior: An analysis of 3350 twin pairs. *Addiction, 93*, 1375–1384.

Engwall, D., Hunter, R., & Steinberg, M. (2004). Gambling and other risk behaviors on university campuses. *Journal of American College Health, 52*, 245–255.

Floyd, K., Whelan, J. P., & Meyers, A. W. (2006). Use of warning messages to modify gambling beliefs and behavior in a laboratory investigation. *Psychology of Addictive Behaviors, 20*, 69–74.

First, M. B., Spitzer, R. L, Gibbon M., & Williams, J. B. W. (2001). *Structured Clinical Interview for DSM-IV-TR Axis I Disorders, Research Version, Patient Edition (SCID-I/P)*. New York: Biometrics Research, New York State Psychiatric Institute.

Gambino, B., Fitzgerald, R., Shaffer, H., Renner, J., & Courtnage, P. (1993). Perceived family history of problem gambling and scores on SOGS. *Journal of Gambling Studies, 9*, 169–184.

Gerstein, D. R., Volberg, R. A., Toce, M. T., Harwood, H., Johnson, R. A., Buie, T., et al. (1999). *Gambling impact and behavior study: Report to the national gambling impact study commission.* Chicago, IL: National Opinion Research Center.

Goudriaan, A. E., Oosterlaan, J., de Beurs, E., & Van de Brink, W. (2004). Pathological gambling: A Comprehensive review of biobehavioral findings. *Neuroscience and Biobehavioral Reviews, 28*, 123–141.

Grant J. E., & Kim, S. W. (2002). Gender differences in pathological gambling disorder. *Psychiatric Quarterly, 73*, 239–247.

Grant, J. E., Kim, S. W., Potenza, M. N., Blanco, C., Ibanez, A., Stevens, L., Hektner, J. M., & Zaninelli, R. (2003). Paroxetine treatment of pathological gambling: A multi-centre randomized controlled trial. *International Clinical Psychopharmacology, 18*, 243–249.

Grant, J. E., Potenza, M. N., Hollander, E., Cunningham-Williams, R., Nurminen, T., Smits, G., & Kallio, A. (2006). Multicenter investigation of the opioid antagonist nalmefene in the treatment of pathological gambling. *American Journal of Psychiatry, 163*, 303–312.

Grun, L., & McKeigue, P. (2000). Prevalence of excessive gambling before and after introduction of a national lottery in the United Kingdom: Another example of the single distribution theory. *Addiction, 95*, 959–966.

Gupta, R., & Derevensky, J. L. (1998). Adolescent gambling behavior: A prevalence study and examination of the correlates associated with excessive gambling. *Journal of Gambling Studies, 14*, 319–345.

Herscovitch, J. (1999). *Alcoholism and pathological gambling: Similarities and differences.* Holmes Beach, FL: Learning Publications.

Hodgins, D. C., Currie, S. R., el-Guebaly, N. (2001). Motivational enhancement and self-help treatment for problem gambling. *Journal of Consulting and Clinical Psychology, 69*, 50–57.

Hodgins, D. C., & el-Guebaly, N. (2000). Natural and treatment assisted recovery from gambling problems: Comparison of resolved and active gamblers. *Addiction, 92*, 805–812.

Hodgins, D. C., Makarchuk, K., el-Guebaly, N., & Peden, N. (2002). Why problem gamblers quit gambling: A comparison of methods and samples. *Addiction Research and Theory, 10*, 203–248.

Hodgins, D. C., Wynne, H., & Makarchuk, K. (1999). Pathways to recovery from gambling problems: Follow-up from a general population survey. *Journal of Gambling Studies, 15*, 93–104.

Holden, C. (2001). "Behavioral" addictions: Do they exist? *Science, 294*, 980–892.

Johnson, E. E., Hamer, R., & Nora, R. M. (1998). The Lie/Bet Questionnaire for screening pathological gamblers: A follow-up study. *Psychological Reports, 83*, 1219–1224.

Johnson, E. E., Hamer, R., Nora, R. M., Tan, B., Eisenstein, N., & Engelhart, C. (1977). The Lie/Bet Questionnaire for screening pathological gamblers. *Psychological Reports, 80*, 83–88.

King, M. P., & Tucker, J. A. (2000). Behavior change patterns and strategies distinguishing moderation drinking and abstinence during the natural resolution of alcohol problems without treatment. *Psychology of Addictive Behavior, 14*, 48–55.

Klingelmann, H. K., Sobell, L., Barker, J., Blomqvist, J., Cloud, W., Ellinstad, T., et al. (2001). *Promoting self-change from problem substance use: Practical implications for policy prevention and treatment.* Boston, MA: Kluwer.

Koepp, M. J., Gunn, R. M., Lawrence, A. D., Cunningham, V. J., Dagher, A., Jones, et al. (1998). Evidence for striatal dopamine release during a video game. *Nature, 393*, 266–268.

LaBrie, J. W., Quinlan, T., Schiffman, J. E., & Earleywine, M. E. (2005). Performance of alcohol and safer sex change rulers compared with readiness to change questionnaires. *Psychology of Addictive Behaviors, 19*, 112–115.

Ladd, G. T., Molinda, C. A., Kerins, G. J., & Perry, N. M. (2003). Gambling participants and problems among older adults. *Journal of Geriatric Psychiatry and Neurology, 16*, 172–177.

Ladd, G. T., & Petry, N. M. (2002a). Disordered gambling among university based medical and dental patients: A focus on internet gambling. *Psychology of Addictive Behavior, 16*, 76–79.

Ladd, G. T., & Petry, N. M. (2002b). Gender differences among pathological gamblers with and without substance abuse treatment histories. *Experimental and Clinical Psychopharmacology, 11*, 202–309.

Ladouceur, R. (2004). Perceptions among pathological and nonpathological gamblers. *Addictive Behaviors, 29*, 555–565.

Ladouceur, R. (2005). Controlled gambling for pathological gamblers. *Journal of Gambling Studies, 21*, 49–57.

Ladouceur, R. (1996). The prevalence of pathological gambling in Canada. *Journal of Gambling Studies, 12*, 129–142.

Ladouceur, R., Bouchard, C., Rheaume, N., Jacques, C., Ferland, F., Leblond, J., et al. (2000). Is the SOGS an accurate measure of pathological gambling among children, adolescents, and adults? *Journal of Gambling Studies, 16*, 1–24.

Ladouceur, R., Boisvert, J. M., Pepin, M., Loranger, M., & Sylvain, C. (1994). Social costs of pathological gambling. *Journal of Gambling Studies, 10*, 399–409.

Ladouceur, R., Sylvain, C., Boutin, C., & Doucet, C. (2002). *Understanding and treating the pathological gambler.* West Sussex, England: John Wiley & Sons.

Ladouceur, R., Sylvain, C., Boutin, C., Lachance, S., Doucet, C., & Leblond, J. (2003). Group therapy for pathological gamblers: A Cognitive approach. *Behaviour Research and Therapy, 41*, 587–596.

Ladouceur, R., & Walker, M. (1996). A cognitive perspective on gambling. In P. M. Salkoskvis (Ed.), *Trends in cognitive and behavioural therapies* (pp. 89–120). New York: John Wiley & Sons.

Lesieur, H. R., & Blume, S. B. (1987). The South Oaks Gambling Screen (SOGS): A new instrument for the identification of pathological gambling. *American Journal of Psychiatry, 144*, 1184–1188.

Lesieur, H. R., & Rosenthal, R. J. (1998). Analysis of pathological gambling. In T. A. Widiger, A. J. Frances, H. A. Pincus, R. Ross, M. B. First, W. Davis, & M. Kline (Eds.), *DSM-IV Sourcebook* (Volume 4; pp. 393–401). Washington, DC: American Psychiatric Association.

Lipinski, D., Whelan J. P., & Meyers, A. W. (in press). Treatment of pathological gambling using guided self-change approach. *Clinical Case Studies.*

Lorenz V. C., & Shuttleworth, D. E. (1983). The impact of pathological gambling on the spouse of the gambler. *Journal of Community Psychology, 11*, 67–76.

Marlatt, G. A. (1985). Relapse prevention: Theoretical rationale and overview of the model. In G. A. Marlatt & J. R. Gordon (Eds.), *Relapse prevention: Maintenance strategies in the treatment of addictive behaviors.* New York: Guilford Press.

Marlatt, G. A. (1998). *Harm reduction: Pragmatic strategies for managing high-risk behaviors.* New York: Guilford.

May, R. K., Whelan, J. P., Meyers, A. W., & Steenbergh, T. A. (2005). Gambling-related irrational beliefs in the maintenance and modification of gambling behavior. *International Gambling Studies, 5*, 155–167.

May, R. K., Whelan, J. P., Steenbergh, T. A., & Meyers, A. W. (2003). The Gambling Self-Efficacy Questionnaire: An initial psychometric evaluation. *Journal of Gambling Studies, 19, 339–357.*

McGinn, L. K., & Sanderson W. C. (2001). What allows cognitive behavioral therapy to be brief: Overview, efficacy, and crucial factors facilitating brief treatment. *Clinical Psychology: Science and Practice, 8*, 23–37.

McNeece, D. (2005). *Chemical dependency: A systemic approach* (3rd ed.). Boston, MA: Allyn and Bacon.

Meyers, A. W., May, R. K., Steenbergh, T. A., & Whelan J. P. (November, 2000). *Guided Self-Change for Problem Gambling.* Paper presented at the Annual Convention of the Association for Advancement of Behavior Therapy, New Orleans, LA.

Miller, W. R. (2000). Rediscovering fire: Small interventions, large effects. *Psychology of Addictive Behaviors, 14*, 6–18.

Miller, W. R., & Rollnick, S. (2002). *Motivational interviewing: Preparing people to change addictive behavior* (2nd ed.). New York: Guilford Press.

Miller, W. R., Zweben, A., DiClemente, C. C., & Rychtarik, R. G. (1992). *Motivational enhancement therapy manual: A clinical research guide for therapists treating individuals with alcohol abuse and dependence.* (Volume 2, Project MATCH Monograph Series). Rockville, MD: National Institute on Alcohol Abuse and Alcoholism.

National Research Council. (1999). *Pathological gambling: A critical review.* Washington, DC: National Academy Press.

Neighbors, C., Lostutter, T. W., Cronce, J. M., & Larimer, M. E. (2002). Exploring college student gambling motivation. *Journal of Gambling Studies, 18*, 361–370.

Oei, T. P., & Raylu, N. (2004). Familiar influence on offspring gambling: A Cognitive mechanism for transmission of gambling behavior in families. *Psychological Medicine, 34*, 1297–1288.

Pallanti, S., Quercioli, L., Sood, E., & Hollander, E. (2002). Lithium and valproate treatment of pathological gambling. *Journal of Clinical Psychiatry, 63*, 559–564.

Pallesen, S., Mitsem, M., Kvale, G., Johnsen, B., & Molde, H. (2005). Outcome of psychological treatments of pathological gambling: A Review and meta-analysis. *Addiction, 100*, 1412–1422.

Petry, N. M. (2003a). A comparison of treatment-seeking pathological gamblers based on preferred gambling activity. *Addiction, 98*, 645–655.

Petry, N. M. (2003b). Validity of the Addiction Severity Index in assessing gambling problems. *Journal of Nervous and Mental Disease, 191*, 399–407.

Petry, N. M. (2005a). *Pathological gambling: Etiology, comorbidity, and treatment.* Washington, DC: American Psychological Association.

Petry, N. M. (2005b). Stages of change in treatment-seeking pathological gamblers. *Journal of Consulting and Clinical Psychology, 73*, 312–322.

Petry, N. M., Ammerman, Y., Bohl, J., Doersch, A., Gay, H., Kadden, R., Molina, C., & Steinberg, K. (2006). Cognitive-behavioral therapy for pathological gamblers. *Journal of Consulting and Clinical Psychology, 74*, 555–567.

Petry, N. M., & Mallya, S. (2004). Gambling participation and problems among employees at a university health center. *Journal of Gambling Studies, 20*, 155–170.

Petry, N. M., & Oncken, C. (2002). Cigarette smoking is associated with increased severity of gambling problems in treatment-seeking gamblers. *Addiction, 97*, 745–753.

Petry, N. M., & Pietrzak, R. H. (2004). Comorbidity of substance use and gambling disorders. In H. R. Kranzler & J. A. Tinsley (Eds.), *Dual diagnosis and psychiatric treatment: Substance abuse and comorbid disorders.* (2nd ed., pp. 437–459). New York: Marcel Dekker.

Potenza, M. N., Leung, H., Blumberg, H. P., Peterson, B. S., Fulbright, R. K., Lacadie, C. M. et al. (2003). An fMRI Stroop task study of ventromedial prefrontal cortical function in pathological gamblers. *American Journal of Psychiatry, 160*, 1990–1994.

Potenza, M. N., Steinberg, M. A., McLaughlin, S. D., Wu, R., Rounsaville, B. J., & O'Malley, S. S. (2000). Illegal behaviors in problem gambling: Analysis of data from a gambling helpline. *Journal of the American Academy of Psychiatry and the Law, 28*, 389–403.

Prochaska, J. O., & DiClemente, C. C. (1986). Toward a comprehensive model of change. In W. R. Miller & N. Heather (Eds.), *Treating addictive behaviors: Processes of change.* New York: Plenum Press.

Prochaska, J. O., DiClemente, C. C., & Norcross, J. C. (1992). In search of how people change: Applications to addictive behaviors. *American Psychologist, 47*, 1102–1114.

Raylu, N., & Oei, T. (2004). The Gambling Related Cognitions Scale (GRCS): Development, confirmatory factor validation, and psychometric properties. *Addiction, 99*, 757–769.

Reuter, J., Raedler, T., Rose, M., Hand, I., Gläscher, J., & Büchel, C. (2005). Pathological gambling is linked to reduced activation of the mesolimbic reward system. *Nature Neuroscience, 8*, 147–148.

Robbins, T. W., & Everitt, B. J. (1999). Drug addiction: Bad habits add up. *Nature, 398*, 567–570.

Rosenthal, R. J. (1989). Pathological gambling and problem gambling: Problems of definition and diagnosis. In H. J. Shaffer, S. A. Stein, B. Gambino, & T. N. Cummngs (Eds.), *Compulsive gambling: Theory, research, and practice* (pp. 101–125). Lexington, MA: Lexington Books.

Saunders, J. B., Aasland, O. G., Babor, T. F., De La Fuente, J. R., & Grant, M. (1993). Development of the Alcohol Use Disorders Identification Test (AUDIT): WHO collaborative project on early detection of persons with harmful alcohol consumption II. *Addiction, 88*, 791–804.

Shaffer, H. J., & Hall, M. N. (1996). Estimating the prevalence of adolescent gambling disorders: A qualitative synthesis and guide toward standard gambling nomenclature. *Journal of Gambling Studies, 12*(2), 193–214.

Shaffer, H. J., & Hall, M. N. (2002). The natural history of gambling and drinking problems among casino employees. *Journal of Social Psychology, 142*, 405–424.

Shaffer, H. J., Hall, M. N., & Vander Bilt, J. (1997). *Estimating the prevalence of disordered gambling behavior in the United States and Canada: A meta-analysis.* Boston, MA: Harvard Medical School Division of Addiction.

Shaffer, H. J., Hall, M. N., & Vander Bilt, J. (1999). Estimating the prevalence of disordered gambling behavior in the United States and Canada: A research synthesis. *American Journal of Public Health, 89*, 1369–1376.

Shaffer, H. J., LaBrie, R., Scanlan, K. M., & Cummings, T. N. (1994). Pathological gambling among adolescents: Massachusetts Gambling Screen (MAGS). *Journal of Gambling Studies, 10*, 339–362.

Shaffer, H. J., Vander Bilt, J., & Hall, M. N. (1999). Gambling, drinking, smoking, and other health risk activities among casino employees. *American Journal of Industrial Medicine, 36*, 365–378.

Skinner, B. F. (1953). *Science and human behavior.* New York: The Free Press.

Slutske, W. S. (2006). Natural recovery and treatment-seeking in pathological gambling: Results of two U.S. national surveys. *American Journal of Psychiatry, 163*, 297–302.

Slutske, W. S., Eisen, S., True, W. R., Lyons, M. J., Goldberg, J., & Tsuang, M. (2000). Common genetic vulnerability for pathological gambling and alcohol dependence in men. *Archives of General Psychiatry, 57,* 666–673.

Slutske, W. S., Jackson, K. M., & Sher, K. J. (2003). The natural history of problem gambling from age 18 to 29. *Journal of Abnormal Psychology, 112*, 263–274.

Slutske W. S., Eisen, S., True, W. R., Lyons, M. J., Goldberg, J., & Tsuang, M. (2000). Common genetic vulnerabilities for pathological gambling and alcohol dependence in men. *Archives of General Psychiatry, 57*, 666–673.

Sobell, L. C., & Sobell, M. B. (1996*). Alcohol Timeline Followback (TFLB) user's manual.* Toronto, Canada: Addiction Research Foundation.

Sobell, L. C., & Sobell, M. B. (2000). Alcohol Timeline Followback (TLFB). In American Psychiatric Association (Ed.), *Handbook of psychiatric measures.* Washington, DC: Author.

Sobell, M. B., Breslin, C. F., & Sobell, L. C. (1998). Project MATCH: The time has come to talk of many things. *Journal of Studies in Alcohol, 59*, 124–125.

Sobell, M. B., & Sobell, L. C. (1993). *Problem drinkers: Guided self-change treatment.* New York: Guilford.

Sobell, M. B., & Sobell, L. C. (2005). Guiding self-change model of treatment for substance use disorders. *Journal of Cognitive Psychotherapy, 19*, 199–210.

Sobell, M. B., & Sobell, L. C. (1998). Guiding self-change. In W. R. Miller & N. Heather (Eds.), *Treating addictive behaviors* (pp. 189–202). New York: Plenum Press.

Sobell, M. B., & Sobell, L. C. (2000). Stepped care as a heuristic approach to the treatment of alcohol problems. *Journal of Clinical and Consulting Psychology, 68*, 573–579.

Spanier, G. B. (1976). Measuring dyadic adjustment: New scales for assessing the quality of marriage and similar dyads. *Journal of Marriage and Family, 38*, 15–28.

Specker, S. M., Carlson, G. A., Edmonson, K. M., Johnson, P. E., & Marcotte, M. (1996). Psychopathology in pathological gamblers seeking treatment. *Journal of Gambling Studies, 12*, 67–81.

Steel, Z., & Blaszczynski, A. (1998). Impulsivity, personality disorders and pathological gambling severity. *Addiction, 93*, 895–905.

Steenbergh, T. A., Meyers, A. W., May, R. K., & Whelan, J. P. (2002). Development and validation of the Gambler's Belief Questionnaire. *Psychology of Addictive Behavior, 16*, 143–149.

Steenbergh, T. A., Whelan, J. P., Meyers, A. W., May, R. K., & Floyd, K. (2004). Impact of warning and brief intervention messages on knowledge of gambling risk, irrational beliefs, and behaviour. *International Gambling Studies, 4*, 3–16.

Stewart, J., & Wise, R. A. (1992). Reinstatement of heroin self-administration habits: Morphine prompts and naltrexone discourages renewed responding after extinction. *Psychopharmacology, 108*, 79–84.

Stinchfield, R. (2000). Gambling and correlates of gambling among Minnesota public school students. *Journal of Gambling Studies, 16*(2–3), 153–173.

Stinchfield, R. D. (2002). Reliability, validity, and classification accuracy of the South Oaks Gambling Screen (SOGS). *Addictive Behaviors, 27*, 1–19.

Stinchfield, R. D. (2003). Reliability, validity, and classification accuracy of a measure of DSM-IV diagnostic criteria for pathological gambling. *American Journal of Psychiatry, 160*, 180–182.

Stinchfield, R. D., & Winters, K. C. (2001). Outcome of Minnesota's gambling treatment programs. *Journal of Gambling Studies, 17*, 217–245.

Substance Abuse and Mental Health Service Administration. (2000). *Enhancing motivation for change in substance abuse treatment*. Treatment improvement protocol (TIP) Series number 35. DHHD Pub No. (SMA) 00-34-60. Washington, DC: U.S. Government Printing Office.

Symes, B. A., & Nicki, R. M. (1997). A preliminary consideration of cue-exposure, response-prevention treatment for pathological gambling behavior. *Journal of Gambling Studies, 13*, 145–157.

Sylvain, C., Ladouceur, R., & Boisvert, J. M. (1997). Cognitive and behavioral treatment of pathological gambling: A controlled study. *Journal of Consulting and Clinical Psychology, 65*, 727–732.

Toneatto, T. (1999). Cognitive psychopathology of problem gambling. *Substance Use and Misuse, 34*, 1593–1604.

Toneatto, T., & Millar, G. (2004). Assessing and treating problem gambling: Empirical status and promising trends. *Canadian Journal of Psychiatry, 49*, 517–525.

Tonigan, J. S. (2003). Project Match treatment participation and outcome by self-report ethnicity. *Alcoholism: Clinical and Experimental Research, 27*, 1340–1344.

Tucker, J. A. (1999). Changing addictive behavior: Historical and contemporary perspectives. In J. A. Tucker, D. M. Donovan, & G. A. Marlatt (Eds.), *Changing addictive behavior: Bridging clinical and public health strategies* (pp. 3–44). New York: Guilford.

Volberg, R. A. (1994). The prevalence and demographics of pathological gamblers: Implications for public health. *American Journal of Public Health, 84*, 237–241.

Volkow, N. D., Fowler, J. S., Wang, G. J., & Swanson, J. M. (2004). Dopamine in drug abuse and addiction: Results from imaging studies and treatment implications. *Molecular Psychiatry, 9*, 557–569.

Wagner, E. F. (2003). Conceptualizing alcohol treatment research for Hispanic/Latino adolescents. *Alcoholism: Clinical and Experimental Research, 27*, 1349–1352.

Walker, M. B., & Dickerson, M. G. (1996). The prevalence of problem and pathological gambling: A critical review. *Journal of Gambling Studies, 12*, 233–249.

Weinstock, J., Whelan, J. P., & Meyers, A. W. (2004). Behavioral assessment of gambling: Psychometrics of a Gambling Timeline Followback. *Psychological Assessment, 16*, 72–80.

Welte, J. W., Barnes, G. M., Weiczorek, W. F., Tidwell, M. C., & Parker, J. (2001). Alcohol and gambling pathology among U.S. adults: Prevalence, demographic patterns, and comorbidity. *Journal of Studies on Alcohol, 62*, 706–712.

Welte, J. W., Barnes, G. M., Weiczorek, W. F., Tidwell, M. C., & Parker, J. (2002). Gambling participation in the U.S.: Results from a national survey. *Journal of Gambling Studies, 18*, 313–338.

Whelan, J. P., May, R. K., Steenbergh, T. A., Meyers, A. W., & Avondoglio, J. (2003). *Psychometric evaluation of the GBQ and the GSEQ with a clinical sample*. Paper presented at the 12th International Conference on Gambling and Risk Taking, Vancouver, BC, Canada.

Wickwire, E., Whelan, J. P., Meyers, A. W., & Murray, D. M. (2007). Environmental correlates of gambling behavior in urban adolescents. *Journal of Abnormal Child Psychology, 35*, 179–190.

Wilson, G. T. (1999). Rapid response to cognitive behavior therapy. *Clinical Psychology: Science and Practice, 6*, 289–292.

Winters, K. C., & Kushner, M. G. (2003). Treatment issues pertaining to pathological gamblers with a comorbid disorder. *Journal of Gambling Studies, 19*, 261–277.

Winters, K. C., Specker, S., & Stinchfield, R. (2002). Measuring pathological gambling with The Diagnostic Interview for Gambling Severity (DIGS). In J. J. Marotta, J. A., Cornelius, & W. R. Eadington (Eds.), *The downside: Problem and pathological gambling* (pp. 143–148). Reno, NV: Institute for the Study of Gambling and Commercial Gaming, University of Nevada.

Winters, K. C., Stinchfield, R., & Fulkerson, J. (1993). Toward the development of an adolescent gambling problem severity scale. *Journal of Gambling Studies, 9*, 63–84.

Wise, R. A. (2004). Dopamine, learning and motivation. *Nature Reviews Neuroscience, 5*, 1–12.

8

Appendices: Tools and Resources

This chapter contains measures and resources that therapists can copy and provide to patients. The measures we include are for the Gambling Timeline Follow-Back (examples of the calendar appeared in Chapter 5), the Gamblers' Belief Scale, and the Gambling Self-Efficacy Scale. In addition we included the Goal Statement form and the five GSCG homework assignments.

Appendix 1: Instructions for Completing the Gambling Timeline Follow-Back

We would like you to remember the details of your gambling over the past six months. It is a challenging task. But it is not as difficult as you might imagine, especially when you use the calendar to help you remember. We have found that calendars are very useful in helping people remember their gambling activity. Please read the instructions and tips below before completing the calendar.

Gambling Calendar

1. Every day on the calendar needs to be completed.
2. On those days that you did not gamble at all, mark a "0" or an "X" in that day's box.
3. For *each* day that you gambled, please give the following information:
   - The type of *gambling* you did.
     - Example: slot machines, poker, roulette, horse track, sports, numbers
   - The amount of *time* spent gambling.
     - Note: This item asks how long did you gamble on this occasion? Put your answers in hours. If you gambled for one hour and a half you would write 1.5.
   - The amount of money you *intend* (wanted) to wager.
     - Note: This means, how much money did you plan to bet during the gambling session. Did you set a limit for how much you would wager? For example, if you went to the casino thinking that you would only gamble $100, then you would write $100 on the calendar.
   - The amount of money *risked*.
     - Note: This means, the total amount of money that is from nonwinnings money that you gambled with during the gambling session. This means you take the dollar amount you walked in with in your pocket and add it to any money withdrawn from an ATM or credit card, any money that you borrowed (from friends, family, or the casino) and that you put into play. For example if you walked into a casino with $100 and then borrowed $200 from a friend, you would write $300 on the calendar for the amount risked.
   - The amount of money *won or lost*.
     - Note: This means the amount of total winnings or losses at the end of the gambling session. Therefore, if you began an evening of gambling with $100 and ended up with $150 when you finished, then you would write +$50 for that day. However, if you ended up with only $75 at the end of the same gambling session you would write -$25 for that day.
   - The number of *standard* alcoholic *drinks* you had while gambling.
     - Because alcoholic beverages vary in their alcohol concentration, it is important when collecting drinking information to agree on what constitutes a "drink." Please report your drinking as the standard number of drinks. One standard drink equals 12 ounces of beer, 4 ounces of wine, or 1 ounce of hard liquor.

Helpful Hints

It may be useful to remember specific times when:
1. You didn't gamble for long periods of time.
2. You gambled in a very regular, scheduled, or consistent way. For example, during January you played poker with friends every Tuesday night.
3. It is helpful to mark on the calendar days that are special such as birthdays, paydays, anniversary, etc.

Information to Record on the Calendar

	Sunday	
Date	1	
Type		What the was type of gambling you engaged in?
Time		How long were you gambling that day?
Intend		How much did you intend to gamble with on that day?
Risked		How much did you actually wager (not including wins)?
Win/Loss		At the end of the day, how much did you end up winning or losing?
Drinks		How many drinks did you have while gambling?

Example Week

	Sunday	Monday	Tuesday	Wednesday	Thursday	Friday	Saturday
Date	1	2	3	4	5	6	7
Type	Poker	X	Lottery	Sports	X	Poker & Blackjack	Golf
Time	2.0		0.25	0.25		3.0	3.0
Intend	200		10	100		500	90
Risked	200		10	100		700	90
Win/Loss	0		-10	200		-400	-30
Drinks	2		0	0		7	0

Sunday	Went to the casino, wanting to gamble $200. I played poker for two hours, bet all $200, and had two drinks. I left the casino with $200.
Monday	I did not gamble on Monday.
Tuesday	I bought five $2 Power Ball lottery tickets. I did not win any money from the lottery tickets. It took me about 15 minutes to purchase my lottery tickets.
Wednesday	I placed a $100 bet with a bookie, on the Super Bowl. I beat the spread and won $200. I spent 15 minutes thinking about whether to bet for or against the Giants.
Thursday	Did not gamble.
Friday	I went to the casino and played poker and blackjack for three hours. I planned to bet up to $500. I gambled away the $500 and then took $200 out from the ATM machine. I had 7 drinks and at the end of the gambling session I had only $300.
Saturday	I played 18 holes of golf with a buddy. We played $5 a hole and I had $60 in my pocket. At the end of 18 holes, I owed him $30. It took us about three hours to play the 18 holes.

This page may be reproduced by the purchaser for clinical use.
From: J.P. Whelan, T.A. Steenbergh, & A.W. Meyers: *Problem and Pathological Gambling*   © 2007 Hogrefe & Huber Publishers

Appendix 2: Gamblers' Beliefs Questionnaire (GBQ)

Directions

Read each of the following statements carefully. Rate to what extent you agree or disagree with each statement by *circling* a number.

1. I think of gambling as a challenge.

1	2	3	4	5	6	7
Strongly agree			Neutral			Strongly disagree

2. My knowledge and skill in gambling contribute to the likelihood that I will make money.

1	2	3	4	5	6	7
Strongly agree			Neutral			Strongly disagree

3. My choices or actions affect the game on which I am betting.

1	2	3	4	5	6	7
Strongly agree			Neutral			Strongly disagree

4. If I am gambling and losing, I should continue because I don't want to miss a win.

1	2	3	4	5	6	7
Strongly agree			Neutral			Strongly disagree

5. I should keep track of previous winning bets so that I can figure out how I should bet in the future.

1	2	3	4	5	6	7
Strongly agree			Neutral			Strongly disagree

6. When I am gambling, "near misses" or times when I almost win remind me that if I keep playing I will win.

1	2	3	4	5	6	7
Strongly agree			Neutral			Strongly disagree

This page may be reproduced by the purchaser for clinical use.
From: J.P. Whelan, T.A. Steenbergh, & A.W. Meyers: *Problem and Pathological Gambling*   © 2007 Hogrefe & Huber Publishers

7. Gambling is more than just luck.

1	2	3	4	5	6	7
Strongly agree			Neutral			Strongly disagree

8. My gambling wins are evidence that I possess skill and knowledge related to gambling.

1	2	3	4	5	6	7
Strongly agree			Neutral			Strongly disagree

9. I have a "lucky" technique that I use when I gamble.

1	2	3	4	5	6	7
Strongly agree			Neutral			Strongly disagree

10. In the long run, I will win more money than I will lose when gambling.

1	2	3	4	5	6	7
Strongly agree			Neutral			Strongly disagree

11. Even though I may be losing with my gambling strategy or plan, I must maintain that strategy or plan because I know it will eventually come through for me.

1	2	3	4	5	6	7
Strongly agree			Neutral			Strongly disagree

12. There are certain things I do when I am betting (for example, tapping a certain number of times, holding a lucky coin in my hand, crossing my fingers, etc.) which increase the chances that I will win.

1	2	3	4	5	6	7
Strongly agree			Neutral			Strongly disagree

13. If I lose money gambling I should try to win it back.

1	2	3	4	5	6	7
Strongly agree			Neutral			Strongly disagree

This page may be reproduced by the purchaser for clinical use.
From: J.P. Whelan, T.A. Steenbergh, & A.W. Meyers: *Problem and Pathological Gambling* © 2007 Hogrefe & Huber Publishers

14. Those who don't gamble much don't understand that gambling success requires dedication and a willingness to invest some money.

1	2	3	4	5	6	7
Strongly agree			Neutral			Strongly disagree

15. Where I get money to gamble doesn't matter because I will win and pay it back.

1	2	3	4	5	6	7
Strongly agree			Neutral			Strongly disagree

16. I am pretty accurate at predicting when a "win" will occur.

1	2	3	4	5	6	7
Strongly agree			Neutral			Strongly disagree

17. Gambling is the best way for me to experience excitement.

1	2	3	4	5	6	7
Strongly agree			Neutral			Strongly disagree

18. If I continue to gamble, it will eventually pay off and I will make money.

1	2	3	4	5	6	7
Strongly agree			Neutral			Strongly disagree

19. I have more skills and knowledge related to gambling than most people who gamble.

1	2	3	4	5	6	7
Strongly agree			Neutral			Strongly disagree

20. When I lose at gambling, my losses are not as bad if I don't tell my loved ones.

1	2	3	4	5	6	7
Strongly agree			Neutral			Strongly disagree

21. I should keep the same bet even when it hasn't come up lately because it is bound to win.

1	2	3	4	5	6	7
Strongly agree			Neutral			Strongly disagree

This page may be reproduced by the purchaser for clinical use.
From: J.P. Whelan, T.A. Steenbergh, & A.W. Meyers: *Problem and Pathological Gambling* © 2007 Hogrefe & Huber Publishers

Appendix 3: Gambling Self-Efficacy Questionnaire

Directions

Listed below are a number of situations or events in which some people experience problems in regards to gambling. Imagine yourself as you are *right now* in each of these situations. Indicate on the scale below how confident you are that you would be able to *control* your gambling behavior. For example: How confident would you be that you could limit the amount of time and money you were going to spend gambling so that it would not cause a problem, if you felt confident and relaxed? Circle *100* if you are 100% confident right now that you could control your gambling behavior; *80* if you are 80% confident; *60* if you are 60% confident. If you are more unconfident than confident, circle *40* to indicate that you are only 40% confident that you could control your gambling behavior; *20* for 20% confident; circle *0* if you have no confidence at all about that situation.

		Not at all confident					Very confident
I would be able to control my gambling:							
1.	If I felt that I had let myself down.	0	20	40	60	80	100
2.	If there were fights at home.	0	20	40	60	80	100
3.	If I had trouble sleeping.	0	20	40	60	80	100
4.	If I had an argument with a friend.	0	20	40	60	80	100
5.	If I felt confident and relaxed.	0	20	40	60	80	100
6.	If I were enjoying myself and I wanted to feel even better.	0	20	40	60	80	100
7.	If I had lost money gambling on one day and felt the urge to go win it back the next day.	0	20	40	60	80	100
8.	If I were at a place where other people were gambling.	0	20	40	60	80	100
9.	If I wondered about my self-control over gambling and felt like testing it.	0	20	40	60	80	100
10.	If I were angry at the way things turned out.	0	20	40	60	80	100
11.	If I were relaxing with a good friend and wanted to have a good time gambling.	0	20	40	60	80	100
12.	If my stomach felt like it was tied in knots.	0	20	40	60	80	100
13.	If I were out with friends "on the town" and wanted to increase my enjoyment.	0	20	40	60	80	100
14.	If I met a friend and he/she suggested that we go gambling together.	0	20	40	60	80	100
15.	If I suddenly had an urge to gamble.	0	20	40	60	80	100
16.	If I wanted to prove to myself that I could bet a few times without losing control.	0	20	40	60	80	100

This page may be reproduced by the purchaser for clinical use.
From: J.P. Whelan, T.A. Steenbergh, & A.W. Meyers: *Problem and Pathological Gambling* © 2007 Hogrefe & Huber Publishers

Appendix 4: Goal Statement

On this form describe your gambling goal for the next 6 months. Do you intend to not gamble at all, or to gamble but only in certain ways and under certain conditions?
My current goal is (check *either* Goal 1 *or* Goal 2):

☐   *Goal 1 NOT TO GAMBLE AT ALL*
      *If you checked this goal – Go to the next page **now.***

OR

☐   *Goal 2 ONLY TO GAMBLE IN CERTAIN WAYS*
      If you checked this goal, please complete the following statements.

1. On the average day when I do gamble, I want to gamble about $_____ and spend about _____ hours gambling.

2. I plan to gamble no more than $_____ and spend no more than _____ hours during the course of any single day. That is my upper limit.

3. Over the course of one month (30 days), I plan to gamble my upper limit of money and time (see 2 above) on no more than _____ days. (If you plan to gamble your upper limit of money or time less than one time per month, check here: ☐).

4. I plan to gamble only under the following conditions:
   _____
   _____

5. I plan not to gamble at all under the following conditions:
   _____
   _____

(Now turn to the next page.)

People usually have several things that they would like to change in their lives. Changing their gambling behavior can be one of those things. You have just described your gambling goal for the next six months. Based on that goal, answer the following two questions:

1. At this moment, how important is it that you achieve your stated goal? (How hard are you willing to work, and how much are you willing to do, to achieve your gambling goal?) Answer this question by writing a percentage from 0 to 100 in the designated space below, using the following scale as a guide:

0%	25%	50%	75%	100%
Not important at all	Less important than most of the other things I would like to achieve	About as important as most of the other things I would like to achieve	More important than most of the other things I would like to achieve	The most important

Write your importance rating (from 0 to 100%) here: _____

2. In the designated space below, indicate how confident you feel at this moment that you will achieve your stated goal. In other words, what is the probability that you will achieve your gambling goal? Use the following scale as a guide:

0%	50%	100%
Not at all confident I will achieve my goal	50/50 chance I will achieve my goal	Totally confident I will achieve my goal

Write your confidence rating (from 0% to 100%) here: _____%

This page may be reproduced by the purchaser for clinical use.
From: J.P. Whelan, T.A. Steenbergh, & A.W. Meyers: *Problem and Pathological Gambling* © 2007 Hogrefe & Huber Publishers

Appendix 5: Exercise 1 – Mount Recovery

Usually, a person's gambling problem doesn't develop overnight, and rarely does it disappear overnight. Occasionally people decide to quit or cut back on their gambling and they never have another problem with it. But that doesn't happen for most people. For the majority of people it takes time and effort to take control of their gambling.

Think about a man who is hiking up a bumpy hill. His goal is to reach the top and he really wants to get there. Most of the time he makes steady progress towards the top. But once in a while he slips or trips and falls down. After falling down he has a couple of choices that he can make. He can say to himself, "I've fallen down so I'll just give up and slide back down the hill." Or he can say, "I've fallen down but I'm going to pick myself up and keep going." Which option do you think he should take? Should he give up and forget about the progress he's already made, or should he pick himself up and keep going?

Overcoming a gambling problem can be compared to hiking up a bumpy hill. You may really want to gain control over your gambling, and most of the time you will make steady progress toward your goal. But along the way you may slip on your path to recovery and gamble or gamble more than you intended. If you do slip, it is important that you pick yourself up as soon as possible. Remember, you don't want to end up sliding all the way down the hill. If you pick yourself up and continue along your recovery path, then eventually you can reach your goal.

In some ways, overcoming a gambling problem also is like dieting. If you are on a diet and you slip and have a big piece of chocolate cake, then you can react in one of two ways:

1. You might think to yourself that your entire diet is ruined and decide there's no point in continuing. If you choose this path, then you would give up and return to your old ways of eating. You would end up forgetting the progress that you have already made, and you wouldn't lose weight.

OR

2. You can think that a slip in your diet is not that big of a deal (sort of like tripping on a hike). Although it slows you down, you can learn from your slip, pick yourself back up, and continue on towards your goal. If this is your attitude, then you can still reach your goal.

What if I gamble too much in the future?

Ideally, you will never gamble too much again. But there's always the possibility that you will slip up and gamble too much. If you do slip, the way that you react is very important. Just like the dieting example, it is important to react to a gambling slip in a certain way.

You should take a look at how far you've come on your climb against gambling and what lies below. Take a deep breath, and continue your climb uphill. If you're prepared to accept the slip as only a temporary setback, and then press on to your goal, you are far more likely to achieve it.

If you let slips get the better of you, and simply give up, you won't get to the top of the mountain. And the next time the climb may be even more difficult.

Treat your recovery as a long-term goal, and accept a slip for what it is – a slip, and nothing else. What counts is getting to your recovery goal. Dips or rocks along the way may slow you down. But they *never* have to *stop* you.

Use the true-false quiz below to see how much you have learned about slips.

TRUE – FALSE QUIZ

Directions: Based on what you have learned about how to respond to a slip in your gambling. Place a T for true or an F for false.

_____   If I slip and gamble more than I intended, I should think about it as a learning experience.

_____   If I slip and gamble more than I intended, I might as well give up on my goal.

_____   If I slip and gamble more than I intended, it means that I don't have the willpower to take control of my gambling.

_____   If I slip and gamble more than I intended, I should try to get my gambling under control as soon as possible.

_____   If I slip and gamble more than I intended, I should not beat myself up over my slip.

YOUR NEXT APPOINTMENT IS SCHEDULED FOR:

_____   _____   _____
Day   Date   Time

Appendix 6: Exercise 2 – Making a Decision About Your Gambling

Thinking About Your Gambling

Ask yourself, *"What will I lose and what will I gain by continuing my current gambling pattern?"* and *"What role does gambling play in my life?"* At some point, you may have received real *benefits* from your gambling – a big win, fun, excitement, or an escape from problems. However, since you are reading this, you are probably thinking about the *costs* of your gambling and beginning to see the benefits in a different light.

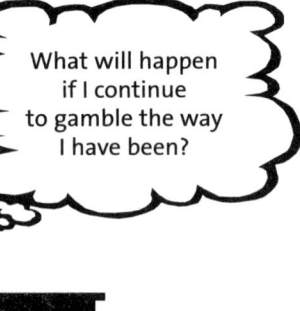

The Decision to Change Exercise – Part 1

Often when we consider making changes in our lives, we don't take the time to carefully examine all sides of the issue. Instead we base our decisions on how we did things in the past or how we feel at the moment. One way to begin to consider changing your gambling is to evaluate the positive and negative sides of it.

Consider these questions about the positive (benefits) and negative (costs) sides of gambling:
Consider these questions:
- What do you like about gambling?
- What social benefits do you get from gambling?
- How is gambling different from other activities?
- Does gambling help you feel better?
- Does gambling solve any of your problems?
- How have your friends and family been affected by your gambling?
- Have much money have you spent on gambling?
- How much time have you spent gambling?
- Have you experienced feelings of depression, guilt or anxiety because of your gambling?
- Have you ever felt controlled by your gambling?

Now it is YOUR TURN. Think about the positives and negatives of gambling.
In the areas below, write down as many of the positives and negatives as you can think of.

Positives of Gambling	Negatives of Gambling

Place a star (*) next to the item that is the most positive aspect of gambling and a star (*) next to the item which is the most negative.

The Decision to Change Exercise – Part 2

Now that you have considered that there are both positive and negative sides to gambling, let's examine what it might take to change. When you are thinking about changing your gambling, it is helpful to think about what your life would be like if: (a) you do change or (b) you do not change your gambling.

Consider these questions about changing your gambling:
- How will my life be different?
- What will I miss if I change?
- What will I lose out on?
- What will I have to do to make a change?
- How will I spend my time instead of gambling?
- How will my family and friends be impacted?
- How will my financial situation change?
- Will changing my gambling impact my health or my job?
- How will I feel about myself if I change?
- How would making a change affect my future?

Now it is YOUR TURN. Think about the positives and negatives of changing your gambling.
In the areas below, write down as many of the positives and negatives of changing your gambling as you can.

Positives of Changing	Negatives of Changing

Place a star (*) next to the item which is the most positive aspect of changing gambling and a star (*) next to the item which is the most negative.

Weighing the Positives and Negatives

Now that you have written down all the positives and negatives of changing your gambling, take a few minutes to compare the list. Think of a balance beam with all the positives of changing your gambling on one side, and all the negatives of changing your gambling on the other. If the negatives and the positives of changing your gambling are about equal, then you have mixed feelings about change and the scale would look like this:

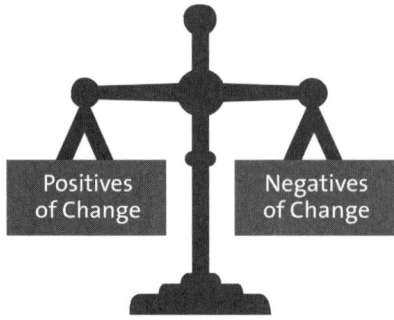

But if you keep adding weights to either side of the scale, then an imbalance will occur.
If the negatives of changing your gambling behavior outweigh the positives then you may NOT be ready to change.

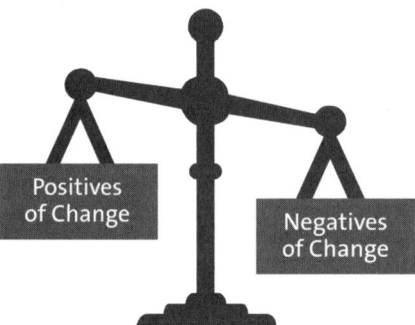

HOWEVER, if the positives of changing outweigh the negatives then you are most likely READY TO CHANGE.

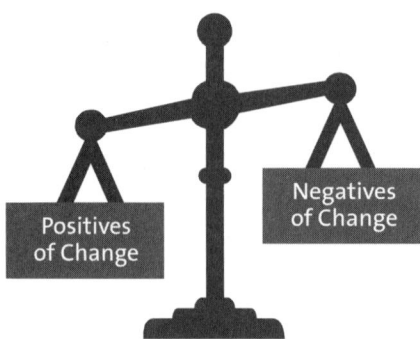

Draw Your Own Change Scale

Now it is YOUR TURN. Compare the positives and negatives of changing your gambling and draw YOUR change scale in the box below to represent the weight of the negatives and positives of changing your gambling. Be sure to label negatives and positives.

WEIGHING THE POSITIVES AND NEGATIVES OF
CHANGING MY GAMBLING

IS IT WORTH IT?

Use the space below to list the three most important reasons why you want to change your gambling.

1. _____

   _____

2. _____

   _____

3. _____

   _____

Appendix 7: Exercise 3 – Understanding Your Gambling Problem

Most people who have problems with gambling have a hard time figuring out what leads them to gamble too much. The first step in changing your gambling behavior is to better understand it. The purpose of this exercise is to help you develop a better understanding of what leads you to gamble too much. It is important that you complete this exercise before your next session because the information you provide here will be used in your next session.

Understanding Your Gambling

An important step towards taking control of your gambling is to *figure out what leads you to gamble*. We don't always act in our own best interest – in the way we think we should – but there are usually reasons why we behave the way we do. Usually the reasons why people gamble fall into two major categories: *triggers* and *consequences*.

Lets first talk about triggers:
Triggers are the things that start you gambling or keep you gambling. They are events that set you up to gamble. These events start you thinking about going to gamble – and sometimes keep you gambling after you should have stopped.
1. *Unexpected Situations:* You're out with friends and they decided to go to a casino for an evening of entertainment. You are on a trip and see signs for a horse track or casino at the next exit. Or you have some unexpected money available.
2. *Situations You Pick:* Going to the casino for dinner or a concert.
3. *Emotional Situations:* You have an argument with someone or a tough day at work. Bumping into an old boyfriend or girlfriend.
4. *Thoughts:* Today you feel lucky. Or, you are depressed, frustrated, or bored and want excitement.
5. *Personal Problems:* You are upset about debts, a fight with your spouse, or an upcoming job interview or court appearance.
6. *Financial Problems:* You have excessive or unexpected bills and gambling seems like the only way to get the money.
7. *Alcohol and/or Drug Use:* After a couple of drinks or a "hit" of a substance you gamble excessively.

As you can see, triggers can be very different. Sometimes a single trigger may set off your heavy gambling and other times it may take many triggers together. To use an extreme example: Learning you need new brakes on your car, you sprained your back, and heard you might be laid off work all in the same week. Those situations together could be a powerful trigger that sets off your gambling. It's rare, of course, that such misfortune would strike all at once, but problem gambling is often proceeded by more than one trigger.

Gambling triggers can be different for everyone. Think about yours. Some gamblers have family problems; others do not. Some may have problems at work; others are happy at their jobs. There are no right or wrong answers that fit every gambler, each one is different. Don't be embarrassed to face or discuss anything you feel is part of your gambling. If it's causing you problems, then we will deal with it.

When thinking about your triggers, it is helpful to remember back to situations when you gamble and try to remember what was going on before you began to gamble. Consider such factors as:
1. Your physical state (were you tired or energetic?).
2. Your emotional state (happy, depressed, etc.).
3. Your thoughts (thinking you're lucky, worried or annoyed about something).
4. The presence of others (friends, relatives).
5. Situations at your job (stress, boredom, etc).
6. Situations at home (fights, difficulties with children).
7. Money situations (large bills due, unexpected income, etc).

Triggers

Write down as many triggers for your gambling as you can think of. *Be as specific as possible.* (Example: Feeling depressed because my spouse is upset, angry, and doesn't talk to me anymore.)

1. _____
2. _____
3. _____
4. _____
5. _____
6. _____

Now let's consider the second major category of reasons why people gamble. These are referred to as *consequences*. These are thoughts, experiences, and results that follow your gambling. Some consequences occur while you gamble (immediate results) and others can occur later (long-term results).

Gambling produces a number of consequences, and some of them are positive. In fact, most people say we gamble to have fun, be entertained, be happy or carefree, ease tension, or forget our problems. Other consequences are very harmful, and it is these harmful results that make gambling a problem.

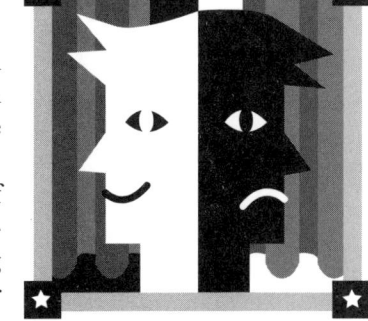

Some gambling *triggers* are directly related to the *consequences*. For example, some people gamble when they are bored (trigger) in order to experience some excitement (immediate result). Yet such gambling can also lead to spending lots of money, which can produce a long-term consequence such as not being able to pay bills.

We sometimes take for granted the *immediate consequences* of gambling, which are usually fairly positive. For some people gambling produces a change in their mood – they change from feeling sad to feeling excited. For others, the immediate consequence of their gambling is just having a good time. It is very important to determine if the immediate results of your gambling are positive, because immediate results usually have a stronger impact on a person's behavior than results that occur later on.

We don't usually think about *long-term consequences* when we are gambling. And later, when we experience the long-term consequences of our gambling, we sometimes don't relate them to the gambling choices that actually caused them. For instance, problems with friends or family may be a long-term result of heavy gambling. However, this long-term consequence may go unnoticed for years because it develops slowly over time. Likewise, a lack of money for bills, household needs, school tuition, or retirement may be a long-term effect of gambling.

So when we speak of the *"consequence"* of a gambling episode, we mean all the combined consequences that occur. We want to look at the overall picture, good and bad. When the consequences are generally more harmful than helpful, a problem exists.

Consequences

Write down as many consequences or results of your gambling as you can think of. When thinking about your consequences, it is helpful to remember back to situations when you gambled and try to remember what happened as a result of your gambling, both immediately and long-term. After you have listed the consequence, tell us whether it is either positive or negative. Be as specific as possible.

(Example: Immediate consequence – I forget all my problems and feel on top of the world while gambling.)

Immediate consequences   **Positive or Negative**

1. _____

2. _____

3. _____

4. _____

Long-term consequences   **Positive or Negative**

1. _____

2. _____

3. _____

4. _____

Appendix 8: Exercise 4 – Dealing With Your Gambling Problem

Now that you've identified the *triggers* and *consequences* related to your gambling, the next step is to learn to use this information to avoid gambling problems in the future. This exercise is intended to help you develop *options*, or alternatives, to excessive gambling.

Please complete this exercise before your next session because the information you provide here will be used in your next session.

Options to Excessive Gambling

When a trigger situation occurs, the desire or urge to gamble becomes strong. There are various ways to respond to these urges – you have *options*. There are four general types of options that you have when the urge to gamble occurs and each has its own consequences (outcomes) associated with it. The next page contains descriptions of the four general types of options.

Options for Trigger and Consequence Situations

Option 1: Gambling Excessively
- This is a very familiar option, and its outcomes are obvious. As you identified in your previous exercise, gambling excessively can produce negative and harmful consequences.

Option 2: Gambling Under Control
- Gambling under control may or may not be a reasonable alternative for you. It involves gambling in limited amounts – in order to avoid harmful results.
- Consider three things when evaluating this option:
  1. How seriously the triggers will affect your gambling. For example, while you may be able to gamble in a controlled manner with friends, you may gamble excessively when alone.
  2. Honestly appraise the triggers and your ability to handle them. Can you gamble in certain situations without it causing problems for you?
  3. The possible consequences you risk by gambling. The more serious the risks, the less likely that controlled gambling is an appropriate option.

Option 3: Not Gambling and Engaging in a Beneficial Activity
- Not gambling is, naturally, a harder course to follow, but it is by far the most beneficial. An example of an alternative activity is going to the movies or talking on the phone with a friend.

Option 4: Not Gambling and Engaging in a Harmful Activity
- Although you refuse to gamble when strong triggers are present, you may behave in other ways that result in equally harmful consequences. For instance, instead of gambling, you may decide to go out and get drunk – for which you later feel guilty.

As you can see, just because a person responds to certain triggers by not gambling, it doesn't mean the results are always positive. Since we've seen that nongambling options can be both "beneficial" and "harmful," it is important to understand these terms. *The "appropriateness" of any option is determined by the consequences it is likely to produce.*

Comparing Options

At this point, having identified the *triggers* and *consequences* related to your gambling, the next step is to decide on the *best options* for you. Some of the *options* might involve things you do, such as visiting a friend, or exercising; others may involve ways of coping, such as learning to deal more effectively with your stress, or to accept things you can't change. The main thing though is to forget about making value judgments at this time. Simply consider all the realistic options that you have.

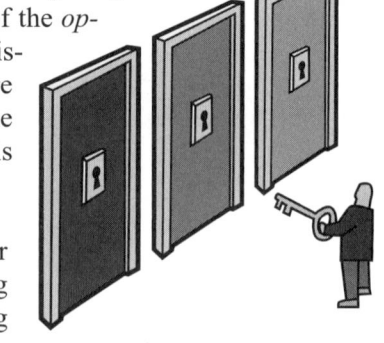

For instance, you may have marital problems. When bickering or fighting occurs, which drives you to gamble, how about considering alternatives such as going to a movie, seeking counseling, talking to a clergyman or clergywoman, discussing the problems with your spouse – or even considering separation or divorce? The options may be simple, or harsh. But the main thing is to consider *all realistic options*. It helps to list them. Once you have developed a list of options, *evaluate them in terms of their overall consequences.* This is where value judgments come in. In evaluating options, it is helpful to ask questions like, "How effective, in the long run, is this option likely to be? What will it take to employ the option? Will it be worth it? And why?"

The final step in choosing your best options is *planning how to use them.* For instance, you may consider:
1. Are you ready to give some of the options a try?
2. Are some easier to implement than others?
3. What personal costs will they involve?

These questions require some serious thought, and it's little wonder why we only tend to consider them when we must.

Now, for each of your trigger and consequence situations you identified in Exercise 3, use one of the options form to describe at least two, and preferably more, *options* to gambling excessively in that situation. Below are guidelines for creating options:
- Be as specific as possible in describing the options.
- All options should be *realistic* – something you can actually do, although you may feel that to putting it into practice might be challenging.

Next, *for each option,* describe the likely *consequences* (what you think would happen if you successfully used that option instead of gambling).
- Be sure to consider *both negative* and *positive* consequences.
- Be sure to consider *both immediate* and *long-term* consequences.

Finally, taking everything into account (for example, the likely consequences, the difficulty of putting the option into practice, your own preferences) indicate at the bottom of the options form which option would be your *first choice* (best option) and which option would be your *second choice* (next best option) for dealing with your trigger and consequences situation.

This page may be reproduced by the purchaser for clinical use.
From: J.P. Whelan, T.A. Steenbergh, & A.W. Meyers: *Problem and Pathological Gambling*   © 2007 Hogrefe & Huber Publishers

Options Form

Trigger Situation # 1 _____

Options and likely consequences: Below, describe at least two, and preferably more, options and their consequences for this trigger.

Option #1 _____
_____

Likely consequences of option _____
_____

Option #2 _____
_____

Likely consequences of option _____
_____

Option #3 _____
_____

Likely consequences of option _____
_____

Select an option for this trigger situation
1. Which option would you select as your *best option*? _____
2. Which option would you select as you *next best option*? _____

Options Form

Trigger Situation # 2 _____

Options and likely consequences: Below, describe at least two, and preferably more, options and their consequences for this trigger.

Option #1 _____

_____

Likely consequences of option _____

_____

Option #2 _____

_____

Likely consequences of option _____

_____

Option #3 _____

_____

Likely consequences of option _____

_____

Select an option for this trigger situation
1. Which option would you select as your *best option*? _____
2. Which option would you select as you *next best option?* _____

Appendix 9: Exercise 5 – Relapse Prevention

Now that you've developed alternatives to your gambling behavior, the next step involves thinking about future high risk situations. This exercise is intended to help you identify those situations that

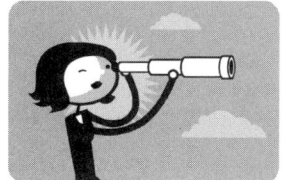

will tempt you to gamble excessively and learn to deal with them more effectively. Understanding when these situations are likely to occur will aid in your process of recovery.

Please complete this exercise before your next session because the information you provide here will be used in your next session.

Use this form to describe options and plans for managing:

High risk situation #1 _____

Option A _____

_____

Option B _____

_____

Action plan _____

_____

High risk situation #3 _____

Option A _____

_____

Option B _____

_____

Action plan _____

_____

High risk situation #3 _____

Option A _____

_____

Option B _____

_____

Action plan _____

_____

This page may be reproduced by the purchaser for clinical use.
From: J.P. Whelan, T.A. Steenbergh, & A.W. Meyers: *Problem and Pathological Gambling* © 2007 Hogrefe & Huber Publishers

Keep Up with the Advances in Psychotherapy!

Stephen A. Maisto, Gerard J. Connors, Ronda L. Dearing

Alcohol Use Disorders

In the series: Advances in Psychotherapy – Evidence-Based Practice

Ocotber 2007, ca. 90 pages, softcover, US $ / € 24.95
(Series Standing Order: US $ / € 19.95)
ISBN: 978-0-88937-317-4

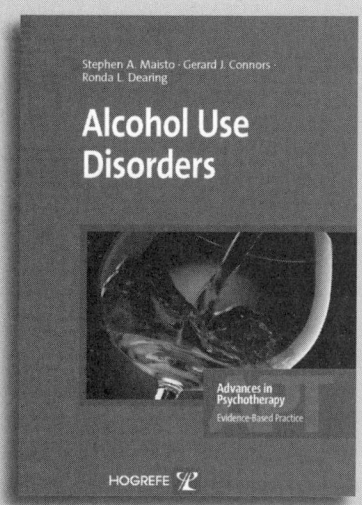

Practice-oriented, evidence-based guidance on treating alcohol problems – one of the most widespread health problems in modern society.

This volume in the series *Advances in Psychotherapy – Evidence-Based Practice* provides therapists and students with practical and evidence-based guidance on the diagnosis and treatment of alcohol problems.

Alcohol abuse and alcohol dependence are widespread, and the individual and societal problems associated with these disorders have made the study and treatment of alcohol use disorders a clinical research priority. Research over the past several decades has led to the development of excellent empirically supported treatment methods. This book aims to increase clinicians' access to empirically supported interventions for alcohol use disorders, with the hope that these methods will become the standard in clinical practice.

Table of Contents

1. Description
1.1. Terminology • 1.2. Definition • 1.3. Epidemiology • 1.4. Course and Prognosis • 1.5. Differential Diagnosis • 1.6. Comorbidities • 1.7. Diagnostic Procedures and Documentation

2. Theories and Models of the Disorder

3. Diagnosis and Treatment Indications

4. Treatment
4.1. Methods of Treatment • 4.2. Mechanisms of Action • 4.3. Efficacy and Prognosis • 4.4. Variations and Combinations of Methods • 4.5. Problems in Carrying out the Treatments

5. Case Vignette

6. Further Reading

7. References

8. Appendix: Tools and Resources

Order online at: **www.hhpub.com** or call toll-free **(800) 228-3749**
please quote "APT 2007" when ordering

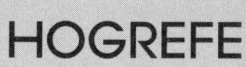

Hogrefe & Huber Publishers · 30 Amberwood Parkway · Ashland, OH 44805
Tel: (800) 228-3749 · Fax: (419) 281-6883
Hogrefe & Huber Publishers · Rohnsweg 25 · D-37085 Göttingen
Tel: +49 551 49 609-0 · Fax: +49 551 49 609-88
E-Mail: custserv@hogrefe.com

Keep Up with the Advances in Psychotherapy!

Stephen W. Touyz, Janet Polivy, Phillippa Hay

Eating Disorders
In the series: Advances in Psychotherapy – Evidence-Based Practice

2008, ca. 90 pages, softcover, US $ / € 24.95
(Series Standing Order: US $ / € 19.95)
ISBN: 978-0-88937-318-1

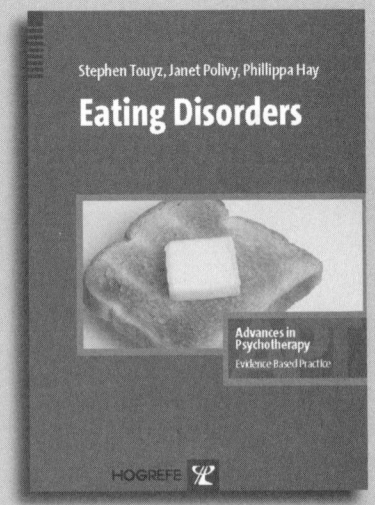

Eating disorders are causing increasing problems in our society, and many approaches to treatment are used, some more successful than others. This volume provides therapists and students with practical and evidence-based guidance on diagnosis and treatment of eating disorders. It builds on existing knowledge as well as the enormous wealth of clinical experience that the authors have developed over the past three decades. It assumes a basic understanding of therapeutic intervention and some clinical training. This book will be of interest not only to those clinicians who have developed a special expertise in eating disorders, but to psychologists, psychiatrists, general practitioners, dietitians, social workers, nurses, and other allied mental health practitioners as well.

Table of Contents
1. Description
1.1. Terminology • 1.2. Definition • 1.3. Epidemiology • 1.4. Course and Prognosis • 1.5. Differential Diagnosis • 1.6. Comorbidities • 1.7. Diagnostic Procedures and Documentation
2. Theories and Models of the Disorder
3. Diagnosis and Treatment Indications
4. Treatment
4.1. Methods of Treatment • 4.2. Mechanisms of Action • 4.3. Efficacy and Prognosis • 4.4. Variations and Combinations of Methods • 4.5. Problems in Carrying out the Treatments
5. Case Vignette
6. Further Reading
7. References
8. Appendix: Tools and Resources

Order online at: **www.hhpub.com** or call toll-free **(800) 228-3749**
please quote "APT 2007" when ordering

Hogrefe & Huber Publishers · 30 Amberwood Parkway · Ashland, OH 44805
Tel: (800) 228-3749 · Fax: (419) 281-6883
Hogrefe & Huber Publishers · Rohnsweg 25 · D-37085 Göttingen
Tel: +49 551 49 609-0 · Fax: +49 551 49 609-88
E-Mail: custserv@hogrefe.com

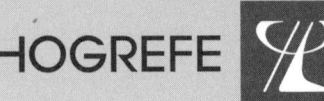

Keep Up to Date with the...

Advances in Psychotherapy – Evidence-Based Practice

Developed and edited with the support of the Society of Clinical Psychology (APA Division 12)

Series Editor: *Danny Wedding*
Associate Editors: *Larry Beutler, Kenneth E. Freedland, Linda Carter Sobell, David A. Wolfe*

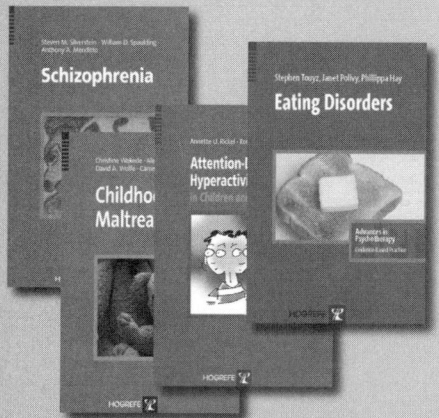

Main features of the volumes:

- **Evidence-based:** Proven, effective approaches to each disorder.
- **Practice-oriented:** Emphasis is on information that is useful in daily practice.
- **Authoritative:** Written and edited by leading authorities.
- **Easy-to-read:** Tables, illustrations, test boxes, and marginal notes highlight important information.
- **Compact:** Each volume consists of 80–120 pages.
- **Regular publication:** We aim to publish 4 volumes each year.

Current & Forthcoming Volumes at a Glance:

- Vol. 1: Bipolar Disorder by *Robert P. Reiser, Larry W. Thompson* (July 2005)
- Vol. 2: Heart Disease by *Judith A. Skala, Kenneth E. Freedland, Robert M. Carney* (August 2005)
- Vol. 3: Obsessive-Compulsive Disorder by *Jonathan S. Abramowitz* (January 2006)
- Vol. 4: Childhood Maltreatment by *Christine Wekerle, Alec L. Miller, David A. Wolfe, Carrie B. Spindel* (July 2006)
- Vol. 5: Schizophrenia by *Steven M. Silverstein, William D. Spaulding, Anthony A. Menditto* (August 2006)
- Vol. 6: Treating Victims of Mass Disaster and Terrorism by *Jennifer Housley, Larry E. Beutler* (October 2006)
- Vol. 7: Attention-Deficit/Hyperactivity Disorder in Children and Adults by *Annette U. Rickel, Ronald T. Brown* (April 2007)
- Vol. 8: Problem and Pathological Gambling by *James P. Whelan, Timothy A. Steenbergh, Andrew W. Meyers* (July 2007)
- Vol. 9: Chronic Illness in Children and Adolescents by *Ronald T. Brown, Brian P. Daly, Annette U. Rickel* (August 2007)
- Vol. 10: Alcohol Use Disorders by *Stephen A. Maisto, Gerard J. Connors, Ronda L. Dearing* (October 2007)
- Chronic Pain by *Beverly J. Field, Robert A. Swarm* (January 2008)
- Social Anxiety Disorder by *Martin M. Antony, Karen Rowa* (February 2008)
- Eating Disorders by *Stephen W. Touyz, Janet Polivy, Phillippa Hay* (2008)
- Borderline Disorder by *Martin Bohus, Kate Comtois* (Publication date t.b.a.)
- Nicotine and Tobacco Dependence by *Alan L. Peterson* (Publication date t.b.a.)
- Depression by *Lynn Rehm* (Publication date t.b.a.)
- Hypochondriasis and Health Anxiety by *Jonathan S. Abramowitz, Autumn Braddock* (Publication date t.b.a.)
- Suicidal Behavior and Self-Injury by *Richard McKeon* (Publication date t.b.a.)

Further Volumes being planned on:

Enuresis and Encopresis • Agoraphobia and Panic Disorder • Male Sexual Dysfunction • Female Sexual Dysfunction • Diabetes

Bibliographic features of each volume: ca. 80–120 pages, softcover, US $/€ 24.95, **Standing order price US $ / € 19.95** (minimum 4 successive vols.)
Special rates for members of the Society of Clinical Psychology (APA D12)
– Single volume: US $19.95 – Standing order: US $17.95 per volume (please supply APA membership # when ordering)

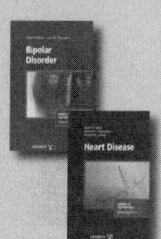

Order online at: **www.hhpub.com** or call toll-free **(800) 228-3749**
please quote "APT 2007" when ordering

Save 20% with a Series Standing Order

Hogrefe & Huber Publishers · 30 Amberwood Parkway · Ashland, OH 44805
Tel: (800) 228-3749 · Fax: (419) 281-6883
Hogrefe & Huber Publishers · Rohnsweg 25 · D-37085 Göttingen
Tel: +49 551 49 609-0 · Fax: +49 551 49 609-88
E-Mail: custserv@hogrefe.com

HOGREFE

Advances in Psychotherapy – Evidence-Based Practice

Developed and edited in consultation with the Society of Clinical Psychology (APA Division 12).

Keep Up with the Advances in Psychotherapy!

Pricing / Standing Order Terms

Regular Prices: Single volume – US $ / € 24.95; Series Standing Order – US $ / € 19.95
APA D12 member prices: Single volume – $19.95; Series Standing Order – $17.95
With a Series Standing Order you will automatically be sent each new volume upon its release. After a minimum of 4 successive volumes, the Series Standing Order can be cancelled at any time. If you wish to pay by credit card, we will hold the details on file but your card will only be charged when a new volume actually ships.

Order Form (please check a box)

[ ] I would like to place a Standing Order for the series at the special price of US $ / € 19.95 per volume, starting with volume no. ....

[ ] I am a D12 Member and would like to place a Standing Order for the series at the special D12 Member Price of US $17.95 per volume, starting with volume no. ......
My APA membership no. is:

[ ] I would like to order the following single volumes at the regular price of US $ / € 24.95 per volume.

[ ] I am a D12 Member and would like to order the following single volumes at the special D12 Member Price of US $19.95 per volume.
My APA D12 membership no. is:

Qty.	Author / Title / ISBN	Price	Total
		Subtotal	
	WA residents add 8.8% sales tax		
	Shipping & handling: USA — US $6.00 per volume (multiple copies: US $1.25 for each further copy) Canada — US $8.00 per volume (multiple copies: US $2.00 for each further copy) South America: — US $10.00 per volume (multiple copies: US $2.00 for each further copy) Europe: — € 6.00 per volume (multiple copies: € 1.25 for each further copy) Rest of the World: — € 8.00 per volume (multiple copies: € 1.50 for each further copy)		
		Total	

[ ] Check enclosed   [ ] Please bill me   Charge my: [ ] VISA   [ ] MC   [ ] AmEx
Card # _____ CVV2/CVC2/CID # _____ Exp date _____
Signature _____
Shipping address (please include phone & fax) _____
_____
_____
_____

Order online at: **www.hhpub.com** or call toll-free **(800) 228-3749**
please quote "APT 2007" when ordering

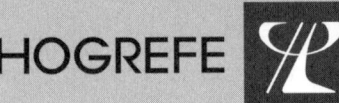

Hogrefe & Huber Publishers · 30 Amberwood Parkway · Ashland, OH 44805
Tel: (800) 228-3749 · Fax: (419) 281-6883
Hogrefe & Huber Publishers · Rohnsweg 25 · D-37085 Göttingen
Tel: +49 551 49 609-0 · Fax: +49 551 49 609-88
E-Mail: custserv@hogrefe.com

HOGREFE